URODYNAMICS

MADE EASY

Fourth Edition

URODYNAMICS

MADE EASY

Christopher R. Chapple, BSc, MBBS, MD, FRCS(Urol), FEBU

Consultant Urological Surgeon, Sheffield Teaching Hospitals, Royal Hallamshire Hospital, Sheffield; Honorary Professor of Urology, University of Sheffield, Sheffield; Visiting Professor of Urology, Sheffield Hallam University, Sheffield, UK

Christopher J. Hillary, MBChB, MRCS, PhD

Specialist Registrar in Urology, Sheffield Teaching Hospitals, Royal Hallamshire Hospital, Sheffield, UK

Anand Patel, MBChB, MRCS, MFPM

Medical Development Director, Global Drug Development, Ipsen, UK

Scott A. MacDiarmid, MD

Director, Alliance Urology Specialists, Bladder Control and Pelvic Pain Center, Greensboro, North Carolina; Clinical Associate Professor, Department of Urology, University of North Carolina, Chapel Hill, North Carolina, USA

Foreword by

Alan J. Wein, MD, PhD(Hon), FACS

Founders Professor of Urology and Director, Residency Program in Urology, Perelman School of Medicine at the University of Pennsylvania, Philadelphia, USA

ELSEVIER

ELSEVIER

First edition 1991
Second edition 2000
Third edition 2009
Fourth edition 2019

The right of Christopher R. Chapple, Scott A. MacDiarmid, Anand Patel, and Christopher J. Hillary to be identified as author of this work has been asserted by them in accordance with the Copyright, Designs and Patents Act 1988.

Notices

Practitioners and researchers must always rely on their own experience and knowledge in evaluating and using any information, methods, compounds or experiments described herein. Because of rapid advances in the medical sciences, in particular, independent verification of diagnoses and drug dosages should be made. To the fullest extent of the law, no responsibility is assumed by Elsevier, authors, editors or contributors for any injury and/or damage to persons or property as a matter of products liability, negligence or otherwise, or from any use or operation of any methods, products, instructions, or ideas contained in the material herein.

ISBN: 978-0-7020-7340-3

Printed in Scotland
Last digit is the print number: 9   8   7   6

Content Strategist: Laurence Hunter
Content Development Specialist: Trinity Hutton
Project Manager: Beula Christopher
Design: Ashley Miner
Illustration Manager: Nichole Beard
Marketing Manager: Deborah Watkins

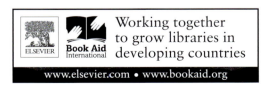

Working together
to grow libraries in
developing countries

www.elsevier.com • www.bookaid.org

Contents

Foreword

The title *Urodynamics Made Easy* may seem like a contradiction in terms, but in this case I can assure you that it is not. This remarkable little treatise, of which I have every edition, each better than its predecessor but about the same size, should be a part of every urology trainee's initial armamentarium and should be in the mini-library of any other generalist or specialist who deals frequently with patients with lower urinary tract (LUT) dysfunction and wonders what the tracings attached to the urology consultation really mean.

There are 10 chapters which concisely describe the basics of the anatomy and neurophysiology of the LUT, the overall clinical evaluation of the patient with LUT dysfunction and the individual urodynamic procedures. The abnormalities seen in storage, emptying and sensory disorders are described and pictured, as well as what might be expected in patients with neurological injury or disease and in those with fibrotic bladders. There is a separate chapter on paediatric issues. Appendices include how to set up and do a study, normal values and sample recordings.

The text is clear and precise, and illustrations are well done and schematically accurate. The biggest compliment any reviewer can pay to a book is to say 'I wish I were an author.' In this case, I do.

Alan J. Wein
Philadelphia, 2019

Preface

This book, which is the fourth edition, once again provides a user-friendly approach to urodynamics as an essential component of the evaluation of the lower urinary tract.

The emphasis of this book is to show the ethos behind the practice of urodynamics and how it needs to be integrated into the evaluation of all patients with lower urinary tract symptoms. It is particularly essential to recognise that *urodynamics* as a term encompasses a whole spectrum of diagnostic approaches, starting with a careful history and incorporating flow rates, residuals and the bladder diary, and of course, where appropriate, progressing on to more invasive techniques, such as pressure flow urodynamics.

It is my hope that this book dispels the myths firstly that urodynamics equates with pressure/flow studies and secondly that the jargon makes the subject unintelligible. If that is the case, then this book will have fulfilled its aim.

This guide outlines the principles and practice of urodynamics in the routine clinical management of patients. Although the 'bladder is an unreliable witness' and is associated with a variety of nonspecific symptoms, improvements in urodynamic techniques and electronic equipment over the past 20 years have allowed the widespread use of objective investigations to clarify these symptoms.

Urodynamics is the study of pressure and flow relationships during the storage and transport of urine within the urinary tract. In routine practice, most urodynamic investigations are focused on the lower urinary tract to:
- investigate bladder filling and voiding function
- accurately define bladder storage disorders
- assess the severity of voiding dysfunction.

Upper tract urodynamics is usually carried out in specialist units.

The first edition of this book was compiled with Tim Christmas, who sadly passed away in 2011. For the second edition, I worked with Scott MacDiarmid, a long-standing friend and colleague working in the United States. Anand Patel joined the last edition of the book and made an enormous contribution. I am now delighted to welcome a new coauthor, Chris Hillary, who has made a very substantive contribution to this edition. It is my hope that you will enjoy reading it.

Christopher R. Chapple, Sheffield

Acknowledgements

We would like to thank the International Continence Society for its permission to reproduce definitions from the latest documents on standardization. We are most grateful to Jen Tidman for her help with the editorial process and to the following companies that kindly provided information on urodynamic equipment, figures and traces for inclusion in this book:

Gaeltec
Glendale Road
Isle of Skye
IV55 8GU
Scotland
http://www.gaeltec.com

Genesis Medical Limited
7 Trojan Business Park
Cobbold Road
London
NW10 9ST
UK
https://www.genmedhealth.com

Laborie Medical Technologies
6415 Northwest Drive
Unit 11, Mississauga
Ontario
L4V 1X1
Canada
http://www.laborie.com

Medical Measurement Systems (MMS)
P.O. Box 580
7500 AN Enschede
The Netherlands
http://www.mmsinternational.com

T-DOC Company, LLC
5 Edgemoor Road
Suite 212
Wilmington, DE 19809
USA
http://www.laborie.com/products/t-doc-air-charged-urodynamic-catheters/

CHAPTER 1

Clinical evaluation of the lower urinary tract

INTRODUCTION

The bladder and the urethra comprise the lower urinary tract and act as a single (vesicourethral) unit during normal lower urinary tract function. The ultimate role of this unit is to convert a continuous process of micturition into an intermittent process of elimination and it therefore has two main functions:

- to store urine (storage)
- to efficiently empty urine (voiding).

If the function of this vesicourethral unit is disturbed, urinary dysfunction along with associated lower urinary tract symptoms (LUTS) may occur. Management of lower urinary tract dysfunction is based on the findings of:

- a detailed history and focused physical examination
- appropriate laboratory studies
- endoscopy and radiography to provide structural information when clinically indicated
- urodynamic studies to provide functional information when clinically indicated.

FOCUSED HISTORY AND PHYSICAL EXAMINATION

First and foremost, an appropriately focused clinical history of the patient's symptoms allows the formation of a working diagnosis, which can help to direct specific clinical questions and subsequent investigations and management. Previously, a plethora of overlapping and confusing terms relating to lower urinary tract dysfunction were in use; however, the International Continence Society (ICS) has published terminology reports to standardize the terms used when describing LUTS, thus enabling consistent and accurate reporting of symptoms, and enabling further investigations and

1

Lower urinary tract symptoms		
Storage	**Voiding**	**Post-micturition**
Urgency	Hesitancy	Feeling of incomplete emptying
Increased daytime frequency	Intermittency	Post-micturition dribble
Nocturia	Slow stream	
Urinary incontinence	Splitting or spraying	
Altered bladder sensation	Straining	
	Terminal dribble	

Table 1.1 *Lower urinary tract symptoms.*

management to be appropriately directed. It is recommended that only standardized terminology be used when describing LUTS.

The ICS has broadly categorized LUTS into three groups (Table 1.1) related to their timing within the bladder (voiding) cycle. The three stages of the bladder cycle are:
1. **storage** – during which passive filling of the bladder occurs
2. **voiding** – during which the vesicourethral unit actively expels the bladder contents
3. **post-micturition** – immediately after a voiding phase, when the bladder returns to a storage function.

Specific definitions for LUTS are listed in the box at the end of this chapter.

The bladder is frequently said to be an 'unreliable witness'. There are several reasons why this statement accurately reflects the situation. First, LUTS are not disease specific, and diverse pathophysiological processes can produce overlapping LUTS. Second, patients express symptoms in different ways, and this is influenced both by what they are experiencing and how they interpret these symptoms. Finally, as clinicians, we all perform a clinical assessment differently and interpret the clinical picture based on our own experience and prejudices.

Clearly, however, a careful history with emphasis on allocating symptoms to the appropriate stage of the bladder cycle is an important starting point. Failure to store urine can be due to overactivity of the bladder, underactivity of the bladder with overflow or weakness of the bladder outlet. Likewise, although voiding symptoms tend to be associated in many people's minds with bladder outflow obstruction (BOO), they can also occur in the context of inefficient bladder emptying.

After taking a careful history and carrying out an appropriate clinical examination, laboratory, endoscopic or radiographic tests should be performed prior to urodynamic assessment as clinically indicated.

URODYNAMIC EVALUATION

Appropriate urodynamic tests can only be interpreted after taking an adequate history with the formulation of specific clinical questions, as the principal aims of the urodynamic assessment are to answer the clinical questions by evaluating the function of the vesicourethral unit. Urodynamics is particularly of benefit in objectively identifying *functional* abnormalities of the lower urinary tract, such as those of urinary incontinence and BOO. However (particularly with video cystometry), it may also assist in identifying *structural* abnormalities, such as a prolapse associated with stress urinary incontinence (SUI), vesicovaginal fistulae, urethral diverticula or upper tract vesicoureteric reflux; in the context of the male patient, it can be useful in demonstrating attenuation of the prostatic urethra in association with prostatic outlet obstruction or confirming the diagnosis of bladder neck obstruction.

The term *urodynamics* encompasses any investigation of lower urinary tract dysfunction from the simple to the sophisticated, including:
- frequency/volume chart (FVC)
- bladder diary
- pad testing
- uroflowmetry with and without ultrasound residual estimation
- pressure/flow studies:
  - cystometry
  - video cystometry
  - ambulatory urodynamics
- urethral pressure studies
- other studies:
  - intravenous urodynamogram
  - ultrasound cystodynamogram.

The most frequently performed tests are FVC/bladder diaries, uroflowmetry and pressure/flow studies.

In general, the term *urodynamics* has become synonymous with pressure/flow studies, with most clinicians referring to either cystometry or video cystometry when they use this term.

URODYNAMICS IN PRACTICE

Urodynamics:
- can only be interpreted in association with a comprehensive history and examination of the patient, where they are valuable adjuncts in the investigation of patients who have lower urinary tract symptoms/lower urinary tract dysfunction
- has become synonymous with pressure/flow studies, with most clinicians referring to either cystometry or video cystometry
- is an objective functional test of bladder and urethral function (and may provide some associated structural information)
- may help indicate the most appropriate therapy.

Indication and interpretation of urodynamics

The information acquired from accurately interpreted and well-performed urodynamic studies can be used to:
- diagnose the underlying cause of the lower urinary tract dysfunction
- characterize the lower urinary tract dysfunction
- formulate treatment strategies
- improve therapeutic outcomes
- educate patients regarding their condition.

An experienced clinician with an understanding of urodynamic techniques should carry out the urodynamic study and should interpret the study in the context of the patient's symptoms. As with all practical skills, there is a learning curve, with the interpretation becoming easier with increasing experience. The authors believe that the true clinical value or 'art' of urodynamics is in applying the objective findings of a well-executed study to the individual patient, taking into consideration subtleties in the history and physical examination that may be clinically important.

LOWER URINARY TRACT SYMPTOMS TERMINOLOGY

It is essential to use standardized terminology when discussing LUTS and the results of urodynamic investigations to allow accurate exchange and comparison of information for clinical and research purposes. The official terminology suggested by the standardization committee of the ICS in 2002 is used throughout this book. The ICS terminology for LUTS is summarized in the following, and the terminology for urodynamic parameters is defined in later chapters. Further information regarding terminology can be found on the ICS website (http://www.ics.org).

TERMINOLOGY: LOWER URINARY TRACT SYMPTOMS

Storage symptoms

Increased daytime frequency: the complaint by the patient who considers that he or she voids too often by day (this term is equivalent to the term *pollakisuria* used in many countries).

Nocturia: the complaint that the patient has to wake at night one or more times to void (each void preceded by and followed by sleep).

Urgency: a sudden compelling desire to pass urine which is difficult to defer.

Urinary incontinence (UI): any involuntary leakage of urine.

Stress urinary incontinence (SUI): involuntary leakage on effort or exertion, or on sneezing or coughing.

Urge(ncy) urinary incontinence (UUI): involuntary leakage accompanied by or immediately preceded by *urgency* (*urge urinary incontinence* is a misnomer because it is urgency that is associated with this incontinence, and we therefore believe that it should be called *urgency incontinence*, not urge incontinence).

Mixed urinary incontinence (MUI): involuntary leakage associated with urgency *and* with exertion, effort, sneezing or coughing (a mixture of UUI and SUI symptoms).

Mixed urinary symptoms: involuntary leakage associated with exertion, effort, sneezing or coughing; combined with urgency but not urge(ncy) incontinence.

Enuresis: any involuntary loss of urine (similar to the definition of UI).

Nocturnal enuresis: loss of urine occurring during sleep (an involuntary symptom, as opposed to nocturia, which is a voluntary and conscious symptom).

Continuous urinary incontinence: the complaint of continuous leakage.

Other types of urinary incontinence: may be situational, such as incontinence during sexual intercourse, or giggle incontinence.

Bladder sensations during storage phase

Normal bladder sensation: aware of bladder filling and increasing sensation up to a strong desire to void.

Increased bladder sensation: individual is aware of an early and persistent desire to void.

Reduced bladder sensation: individual is aware of bladder filling but does not feel a definite desire to void.

Absent bladder sensation: individual reports no sensation of bladder filling or desire to void.

Nonspecific bladder sensation: individual reports no specific bladder sensation but may perceive bladder filling as abdominal fullness or spasticity (most frequently seen in neurological patients).

Continued

5

Voiding symptoms

Slow stream: the perception by the individual of reduced urine flow, usually compared to previous performance or in comparison to others.

Splitting or spraying: description of the urine stream (as split or spraying rather than a single discrete stream).

Hesitancy: difficulty in initiating micturition, resulting in a delay in the onset of voiding after the individual is ready to pass urine.

Intermittent stream (intermittency): urine flow which stops and starts, on one or more occasions, during micturition.

Straining: the muscular effort used to either initiate, maintain or improve the urinary stream.

Terminal dribble: a prolonged final part of micturition, when the flow has slowed to a trickle/dribble (compare to post-micturition dribble).

Post-micturition symptoms

Feeling of incomplete emptying: a feeling experienced by the individual after passing urine.

Post-micturition dribble: the involuntary loss of urine immediately after an individual has finished passing urine, usually after leaving the toilet in men or after rising from the toilet in women (compare to terminal dribble).

Other symptoms

Symptoms associated with sexual intercourse: examples include dyspareunia, vaginal dryness and incontinence (should be described as fully as possible – it is helpful to define urine leakage as follows: during penetration, during intercourse or at orgasm).

Symptoms associated with pelvic organ prolapse: examples include 'something coming down', low backache, vaginal bulging sensation and dragging sensation (may need to digitally replace the prolapse to defaecate or micturate).

Genital and lower urinary tract pain: pain, discomfort and pressure may be related to bladder filling or voiding, or may be felt after micturition or even be continuous. The terms *strangury*, *bladder spasm* and *dysuria* are difficult to define and of uncertain meaning, and they should not be used unless a precise meaning is stated. *Dysuria* literally means 'abnormal urination'. However, it is often incorrectly used to describe the stinging/burning sensation characteristic of a urinary tract infection (UTI).

Painful bladder syndrome symptoms

Bladder pain syndrome/painful bladder syndrome/interstitial cystitis (BPS/PBS/IC): suprapubic pain related to bladder filling and associated with other lower urinary tract symptoms, usually increased frequency (but not urgency; diagnosed only in the absence of UTI or other obvious pathology). This is a specific diagnosis usually confirmed by typical cystoscopic and histological features.

CHAPTER 2

Basic structure, function and control of the lower urinary tract

INTRODUCTION

The urinary tract consists of two distinct and mutually dependent components:

- upper tract – comprising the kidneys and ureters
- lower tract – comprising the urinary bladder and urethra.

These components provide a highly sophisticated system of conduits and a reservoir that converts the continuous involuntary production of urine by the kidneys into the intermittent, consciously controlled voiding of urine (micturition at a convenient time and place).

A thorough understanding of the structure, function and control of the lower urinary tract is vital for the accurate interpretation of urodynamic investigations.

THE KIDNEYS AND URETERS

Both kidneys continuously produce greater than 0.5 mL of urine per kilogram of body weight per hour (i.e. >35 mL per hour in a 70-kg man) when functioning properly and adequately hydrated. This urine empties into the kidney's collecting systems, which drain via the ureters.

The ureters function as low-pressure distensible conduits with intrinsic peristalsis, which transport urine from the kidneys to the bladder. The urine drains into the bladder at the vesico-ureteric junction at the termination of each ureter. If correctly functioning, each junction only permits antegrade urinary flow and contains a mechanism to prevent retrograde transmission of urine back into the ureters from the bladder. This serves to protect the upper tract from the high pressures encountered within the bladder during voiding and to prevent infection entering the upper tracts, mechanisms that can become compromised in patients with a neuropathic bladder.

THE URINARY BLADDER

The bladder is a hollow, muscular organ. It has two main functions:

- low-pressure *storage* of urine
- *expulsion* of urine at an appropriate time and place.

Histologically, the bladder is composed of four distinct layers (Fig. 2.1):

1. **Urothelium** – an innermost lining composed of transitional cell epithelium providing an elastic barrier that is impervious to urine and which has a high metabolic rate and an important role in the control of bladder function, whose cells can release several pharmacologically active neurotransmitters.

Fig. 2.1 *Structure of the bladder wall.* *The bladder wall is composed of four distinct layers and includes highly metabolically active urothelial and suburothelial layers. TC, Transitional cell epithelium; LP, lamina propria; CT, loose connective tissue; DM, detrusor muscle; Se, serosa.*

2. **Lamina propria** – this lies immediately beneath the urothelium and superficial to a layer of **loose connective tissue**. It demonstrates high metabolic activity and acts in concert with the urothelium to subserve a key afferent role. Interstitial cells pass through this layer between the urothelium and the underlying detrusor muscle.
3. **Detrusor muscle** – a smooth muscle layer, comprising a functional syncytium of interlacing muscle bundles with fibres running in all directions.
4. **Serosa** – an outer adventitial connective tissue layer.

The base of the bladder extends circumferentially from the ureteric orifices. This region contains the trigone, which is a small triangular muscular area between the two ureteric orifices and the bladder neck and contains a complex plexus of nerves. Above the ureteric orifices is the main body of the bladder.

THE URETHRA AND SPHINCTERIC MECHANISMS

The urethra has two main functions:
1. to provide an effective continence mechanism for the majority of the time (storage phase)
2. to allow adequate bladder emptying with a minimum of resistance (voiding phase).

A further role of the urethra, which seems likely but remains hypothetical, is to provide afferent feedback, which may have important implications in influencing bladder function. The innermost mucosal layer in both sexes is organized in longitudinal folds and during the storage phase when the urethra is 'closed'; this appears in a stellate configuration on cross section. Such a configuration allows significant distensibility, which is necessary during urethral 'opening'.

The submucosal layer contains a vascular plexus which may be involved in improving the seal of a 'closed urethra' by transmitting the tension of the urethral muscle to the mucosal folds.

Apart from the obvious anatomical differences, there are important differences in the configuration of the sphincter mechanisms between males and females (Fig. 2.2).

Table 2.1 contrasts the longer urethra, a prostate and two powerful sphincter mechanisms in the male compared to the single weaker intrinsic sphincter mechanism with a weaker bladder neck and a shorter urethra in the female.

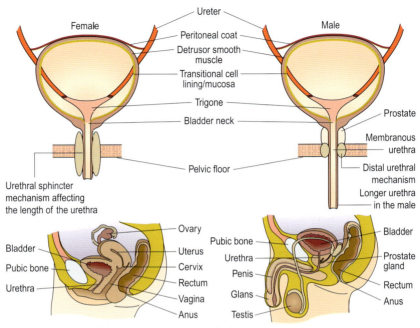

Fig. 2.2 *Anatomy of the lower urinary tract in both sexes.*

Comparison of male and female sphincteric mechanisms		
	Male	**Female**
Proximal bladder neck mechanism	Powerful	Weak
Distal urethral mechanism/ urethral sphincter mechanism (in the female)	Powerful	Prone to the effect of exogenous influences such as pelvic floor weakness and damage or denervation consequent upon childbirth
Prostate	Further increases bladder outlet resistance	Not present
Urethra	Long	Short (3–4 cm)

Table 2.1 *Comparison of male and female sphincteric mechanisms.* This shows why females are much more likely to develop an incompetent urethral mechanism and be prone to urinary incontinence from intrinsic sphincter deficiency.

Male sphincteric mechanisms

In the male, there are two important sphincteric mechanisms:
1. a proximal 'bladder neck mechanism'
2. a distal urethral mechanism at the apex of the prostate.

The proximal sphincter in the male bladder neck provides a powerful mechanism in both maintaining urinary continence and preventing retrograde ejaculation of semen during sexual activity. In patients with a damaged distal urethral sphincter (e.g. a pelvic fracture urethral distraction defect), continence can be maintained solely by the proximal bladder neck mechanism. Ultrastructurally, the bladder neck mechanism consists of a powerful inner layer of muscle bundles arranged in a circular orientation.

The distal sphincteric mechanism is also extremely important, as evidenced by its ability to maintain continence even when the proximal bladder neck mechanism has been rendered totally incompetent by surgical bladder neck incision or a prostatectomy. It is confined to the 3- to 5-mm thickness of the wall of the membranous urethra from the level of the verumontanum down to the distal aspect of the membranous urethra. It is predominantly composed of extrinsic striated muscle, which is capable of the sustained contraction necessary for continence, and to a lesser degree by intrinsic smooth muscle.

Prostate gland

The prostate is made up of smooth muscle and glandular tissue, with the proportion of smooth muscle being increased in benign prostatic hyperplasia. The prostatic smooth muscle is controlled by the sympathetic nervous system, using noradrenaline as the neurotransmitter to act upon α1a-adrenoceptors located on the smooth muscle cells; the resulting contraction increases the bladder outlet resistance and further aids continence in the male.

Female sphincteric mechanisms

Females are much more likely to suffer from urinary incontinence that is due to intrinsic sphincter deficiency than males because of the much less powerful sphincteric mechanism of the female urethra. The bladder neck is a far weaker structure than in the male and is often incompetent, even in nulliparous young women. The bladder neck is also poorly defined, with the muscle fibres having a mainly longitudinal orientation.

Urinary continence is usually reliant on the integrity of the urethral sphincteric mechanism, which like the male distal mechanism is composed of a longitudinal intrinsic urethral smooth muscle and a larger extrinsic striated muscle component. This sphincter extends throughout the proximal two-thirds of the urethra, being most developed in the middle one-third. Damage to the sphincter or its innervation (particularly the pudendal nerve) by obstetric trauma reduces the effectiveness of this mechanism and predisposes to stress urinary incontinence.

Pelvic floor muscles

In females the pelvic floor muscles also have an important role in maintaining continence. The pelvic floor is composed primarily of the levator ani muscle group, the endopelvic fascia and the supporting ligaments. The pelvic organs are maintained in the correct position by this pelvic floor. These tissues form a supporting 'hammock' beneath the urethra; during increases in intraabdominal pressure (e.g. coughing, sneezing), the urethra is compressed against this hammock, thereby keeping the urethra closed and the patient continent (Fig. 2.3).

Failure of this mechanism can cause both descent (prolapse) (Fig. 2.4) and hypermobility of the bladder neck and is an important cause of stress urinary incontinence (see Chapter 5).

FUNCTION OF THE LOWER URINARY TRACT

The function of the lower urinary tract can be split into two distinct phases:
1. the storage (filling) phase
2. the voiding phase.

More than 99% of the time, the lower urinary tract will be in the storage phase, whilst less than 1% of time is spent voiding.

Storage phase

During the storage phase the bladder is filled with urine from the ureters. The bladder needs to accommodate the increase in volume without an appreciable rise in bladder (intravesical) pressure. This receptive relaxation property is called the *compliance* of the bladder. Factors that contribute to compliance are:
- the passive elastic properties of the tissues of the bladder wall
- the intrinsic ability of smooth muscle to maintain a constant tension over a wide range of stress
- the neural reflexes that control detrusor tension during bladder filling.

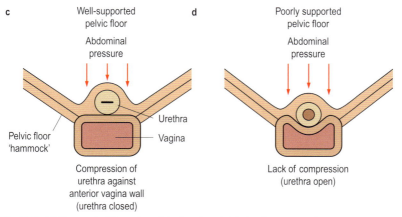

Fig. 2.3 *Midline sagittal illustration of the female pelvis (**a**) with corresponding magnetic resonance imaging scan (**b**) well supported pelvic floor (hammock) (**c**), loss of pressure transmission on the urethra (**d**).*

During the storage phase the urethra and sphincteric mechanisms should be closed, thereby maintaining a high outlet resistance and continence.

Voiding phase

During the voiding phase the reverse activity to that seen during the storage phase must occur. The bladder must cease to relax and instead contract, with

Fig. 2.4 *Prolapse of the bladder neck.* The prolapsing bladder is clearly visible.

synchronous opening of the urethra and sphincter mechanism to decrease the outlet resistance to allow passage of urine. Voiding should be efficient such that there should be minimal or no urine remaining in the bladder at the end of the voiding phase.

During voiding:

1. Urethral relaxation precedes detrusor contraction.
2. Simultaneous relaxation of the pelvic floor muscles occurs.
3. 'Funnelling' of the bladder neck occurs to facilitate flow of urine into the proximal urethra.
4. Detrusor contraction occurs to forcefully expel urine.

URODYNAMICS IN PRACTICE

Storage phase

- The bladder fills passively – detrusor muscle is relaxed.
- Urethral sphincter mechanisms are 'closed' – urethral and pelvic floor muscles are contracted.

Voiding phase

- The bladder actively expels urine under conscious voluntary control – detrusor muscle is contracting.
- Urethral sphincter mechanisms are 'open' – urethral and pelvic floor muscles are relaxed.

Return to storage phase

At the end of voiding the proximal urethra is closed in a retrograde fashion, thus milking back the urine into the bladder. This 'milkback' is seen during contrast studies of the lower urinary tract when the patient is asked to stop voiding. Following this, the bladder returns to a state of receptive relaxation.

NEURONAL CONTROL OF THE LOWER URINARY TRACT

Control of the lower urinary tract is executed via a complex series of peripheral and central neuronal pathways. These pathways:
- coordinate the activities of the bladder and the urethral/sphincter mechanisms
- control receptive relaxation of the bladder (compliance)
- sense bladder fullness
- maintain continence with increasing fullness of the bladder
- initiate voluntary voiding.

Motor (efferent) control

- The storage phase is predominantly under sympathetic control.
- The voiding phase is predominantly under parasympathetic control.

The peripheral innervation of the lower urinary tract is principally from three groups of nerves (Fig. 2.5 and Table 2.2):
1. hypogastric
2. pelvic
3. pudendal.

Sensory (afferent) control

Afferent signalling from the lower urinary tract also occurs along the hypogastric, pelvic and pudendal nerves. These nerves transmit information regarding the fullness of the bladder and the presence of any noxious (chemical or cold) stimuli.

Afferent signalling is involved in:
- involuntary reflexes
- conscious sensation of bladder fullness.

In certain neurogenic or inflammatory conditions, there is upregulation of some of these afferent nerves, causing bladder pain; it is thought that type C

15

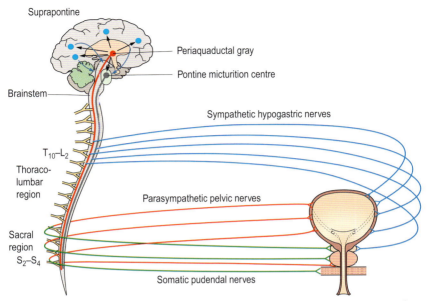

Suprapontine

Periaquaductal gray

Pontine micturition centre

Brainstem

Sympathetic hypogastric nerves

T_{10}–L_2

Thoraco-lumbar region

Parasympathetic pelvic nerves

Sacral region S_2–S_4

Somatic pudendal nerves

Fig. 2.5 *Neural control of the lower urinary tract.* *The somatic, sympathetic and parasympathetic peripheral nerves are shown; the pontine micturition centre, the periaqueductal gray and the suprapontine areas involve the control of storage and voiding of urine. There are extensive interactions at all levels (not shown).*

The principal innervations of the lower urinary tract

	Type	Origin	Detrusor muscle	Sphincteric muscle	Principal neurotransmitter
Hypogastric	Sympathetic	T10–L2	Relaxes	Contracts sphincteric smooth muscle	Noradrenaline
Pelvic	Parasympathetic	S2–S4 (spinal micturition centre)	Contracts	Relaxes	Acetylcholine
Pudendal	Somatic	S2–S4 (Onuf's nucleus)	N/A	Contracts sphincteric striated muscle and pelvic floor	Acetylcholine

Table 2.2 *Principal innervations of the lower urinary tract.* N/A, Not applicable.

afferent nerve fibres are implicated in the involuntary stimulation of detrusor contractions (detrusor overactivity).

Involuntary storage reflexes

Several involuntary reflexes exist, which are mainly located in the lumbosacral spinal cord. With increasing bladder fullness, these reflexes will increase sympathetic activity and inhibit parasympathetic activity, and activate the pudendal (somatic) neurones. These reflexes therefore enhance storage by relaxing the bladder and maintain continence by increasing both intrinsic and extrinsic sphincter tone (guarding reflex).

Voiding reflexes are not confined to the spinal cord, and there are many supraspinal reflexes involved in coordinating lower urinary tract activity that have been discovered in experimentally produced high spinal cord transections.

Desire to void

After infancy, voluntary control of voiding is achieved, which therefore allows voiding to be initiated only in appropriate circumstances. To achieve this, information regarding bladder fullness must be sent to the brain; at an appropriate situation to void the brain must override the peripheral storage reflexes and 'switch' the lower urinary tract into the voiding phase.

Once a threshold level of fullness has been achieved (which will depend on local circumstances and vary between individuals), there will be increasing afferent activity emanating from sensory neurones in the suburothelial plexus of nerves associated with the bladder wall. Parasympathetic afferents in the pelvic nerve will communicate this activity via the spinal cord to the periaqueductal gray (PAG) area in the midbrain. The bladder-filling information is processed at the PAG, and from here the signals are sent to the pontine micturition centre (PMC) in the brainstem and the suprapontine areas of the brain.

The suprapontine areas of the brain comprise the frontal cortex, the hypothalamus, the paracentral lobule, the limbic system and the cingulate gyrus. These are important in the conscious and unconscious control of the PMC. They have a role in delaying micturition, inhibiting premature detrusor contractions and initiating voiding at an appropriate time.

Voluntary control of voiding

The PMC is an essential control centre in the coordination of the voiding process and is itself under the control of the suprapontine area.

If the bladder is sensed to be full but it is inappropriate to void, the PMC will send descending signals to inhibit parasympathetic activity, increase sympathetic tone and increase the pudendal somatic activity to contract the urethral sphincter mechanism and pelvic floor muscles. These mechanisms voluntarily 'tighten up' the bladder outlet and thus maintain continence until an appropriate time and place is found to void.

If the bladder is sensed to be full and it is appropriate to void, the PMC will 'switch' the lower urinary tract into the voiding phase by the release of descending signals to increase parasympathetic activity and inhibit sympathetic and somatic activity.

Once voiding is initiated, secondary reflexes in the urethra, which are activated by urine flow, further facilitate bladder emptying.

Neuronal interactions

The account of the neuronal control of the lower urinary tract given previously is a simplification; extensive interactions exist between the neuronal populations at all levels in the peripheral, spinal and higher central areas. These complex neuronal interactions have led to much controversy regarding the motor control of the lower urinary tract and more recently regarding the sensory feedback. In particular, the role of the suburothelial layer in the processing of mechanosensitive afferents during stretch, which involves a variety of neurotransmitters, is currently the focus of much research. In recent years it has been recognized that stretch of the urothelium can also lead to the nonneuronal release of several mediators, such as acetylcholine, nitric oxide and adenosine triphosphate. In addition, an important group of cells called *interstitial cells* has also been identified, and these undoubtedly have an important role in the coordination of lower urinary tract function. Our understanding of the mechanisms involved is evolving with the continuing research into the mechanisms underpinning lower urinary tract function. Many questions remain to be answered, but it is increasingly clear that the sensory mechanisms are the principal target of contemporary pharmacotherapy and neuromodulatory treatment (e.g. sacral neuromodulation and posterior tibial nerve stimulation).

CONCLUSIONS

A broad understanding of lower urinary tract function and its control is vital to accurately interpret urodynamic investigations and to understand the pathophysiology and treatment of urinary tract disorders such as incontinence, bladder outflow obstruction and neurogenic dysfunction.

CHAPTER 3

Urodynamic procedures

INTRODUCTION

Symptomatic evaluation of urinary tract dysfunction is difficult since the bladder often proves to be an 'unreliable witness', not only because of subjective bias from both the patient and the clinician but also because there is considerable overlap between the symptoms that occur from different disorders. Urodynamic techniques are objective investigations developed to clarify these symptoms. The term *urodynamics* encompasses a variety of complementary techniques of varying complexity (Table 3.1).

In this chapter the indications and methodology for these various techniques will be discussed, along with introducing common clinical findings. Most invasive urodynamic investigations are pressure/flow studies, and these will be discussed in detail in Chapter 4. More detailed discussion of common lower urinary tract disorders and associated urodynamic findings is provided in later chapters.

INDICATIONS FOR URODYNAMIC ASSESSMENTS

Only a good understanding of the various techniques, including their methodology, limitations and specific indications, will allow the clinician to choose an appropriate test. In many cases, several investigations may be necessary to answer all clinical questions, or further investigations may be required if the first investigation was unhelpful or presents a new avenue for investigation.

Before embarking on any urodynamic investigation, the following should be considered:
- Is there a clear indication for the chosen test?
  - Will it aid in diagnosis?
  - Will it aid in making management decisions or assist in patient counselling?

Urodynamic techniques	
Complexity of technique	**Technique**
Simple – voiding diary	Micturition/time chart
	Frequency/volume chart
	Bladder diary
Simple – investigation	Pad testing
	Uroflowmetry ± ultrasound residual
	Ultrasound cystodynamography
	Intravenous urodynamography
Pressure/flow studies (see Chapter 4)	Cystometry
	Leak point measurements
	Video urodynamics
	Ambulatory urodynamics
Complex – investigation	Urethral pressure measurement
	Neurophysiological investigation
	Upper tract urodynamics
	(Whitaker test)

Table 3.1 *Urodynamic techniques.*

- Is this the most appropriate test?
  - Would a simpler test answer the clinical questions?
  - Is a more complex test more likely to answer *all* clinical questions?
- Are there appropriate local facilities and expertise to perform the chosen test?
- Is the most appropriate person, with an understanding of the patient's individual condition, performing the test?

STANDARDIZATION AND QUALITY CONTROL

All urodynamic assessments should be performed in a standardized manner; this not only maintains the quality of the data but also allows for comparison of the results if a patient has a repeat investigation. In addition, a standardized technique and accurate recording of the data using recognized terminology allow the accurate exchange and comparison of information for both clinical and experimental purposes. The official terminology suggested by the International Continence Society (ICS) is used throughout this book. However, investigations must be tailored to individual patients so that the clinical questions are answered thoroughly without undue time spent on obtaining clinically irrelevant data.

Maintaining the quality of any study also requires that all equipment is appropriately set up and regularly calibrated by an investigator with sufficient working knowledge to 'troubleshoot' any problems encountered during an investigation.

In all cases, precise measurement and complete documentation must be coupled with accurate analysis and critical reporting of the results. However, it must be borne in mind that whilst these are objective tests that can be standardized to a high degree, there remains a significant subjective element in the interpretation of the results. Urodynamics is not an exact science!

AIMS OF URODYNAMIC INVESTIGATIONS

The principal aim of any urodynamic assessment is to reproduce the patient's symptoms whilst obtaining physiological measurements to determine the pathophysiology underlying these symptoms.

Both the precise nature of the condition and the severity can be established, thus allowing the clinician to understand the clinical implications and plan further appropriate management.

URODYNAMICS IN PRACTICE

Aims of urodynamic investigations
- Reproduce the patient's symptoms.
- Answer specific clinical questions.
- Establish a precise diagnosis.
- Determine the severity of the condition.
- Plan further investigations or therapies.

In most cases the indications for a urodynamic investigation are clear, and their appropriate application is essential to the modern practice of urology, gynaecology and any specialties dealing with the management of lower urinary tract dysfunction.

CLINICAL NOTES

Always exclude urinary tract infections prior to a urodynamic investigation
- Urinary tract infections (UTIs) are a common cause of lower urinary tract symptoms (LUTS).
- A UTI may aggravate preexisting LUTS.

Continued

- The presence of a UTI may invalidate the results of a urodynamic investigation, as a UTI may falsely result in:
  - ○ increased bladder sensation (± pain or discomfort)
  - ○ detrusor overactivity
  - ○ poor bladder compliance.
- Prophylactic antibiotics may play a role in patients with recurrent UTIs, allowing the study to be performed when the urine is sterile or the patient is asymptomatic.

VOIDING DIARIES

Voiding diaries are the simplest of all urodynamic assessments, yet their value is often overlooked. They provide an important natural urodynamic record of bladder function.

Indications and aims

Voiding diaries are simple, noninvasive tools which frequently form part of the initial evaluation of patients complaining of lower urinary tract symptoms (LUTS), particularly those who have storage symptoms such as increased urinary frequency, incontinence or nocturia.

Voiding diaries give an indication of the voiding pattern and the severity of symptoms, and they add objectivity to the history. They may also give an indication of the impact on the patient's life and may highlight 'coping strategies' that the patient has adopted to help manage symptoms. Voiding diaries are also useful in identifying pathophysiology of renal origin such as abnormal production of urine related to the circadian rhythm.

Several different diaries have been defined by the ICS:

- **Micturition time chart** – records only the times that voids occur with no volumetric data
- **Frequency/volume chart (FVC)** – records the time and volume of each micturition
- **Bladder diary** – records the time and volume of each micturition and may also include other data such as incontinence episodes, pad usage, fluid intake and urgency (Table 3.2).

Method and standardization

The patient is asked to record as accurately as possible the time of events such as voiding activities and any incontinence episodes on the chart and to measure the volume voided using a graduated container. The patient is

Bladder diary

Week commencing:

	Monday		Tuesday		Wednesday		Thursday		Friday		Saturday		Sunday	
	In	Out	In	Out	In	Out	In	Out	In	Out	In	Out	In	Out
6 am	300				350						200		190	
7 am			200				250		350		100			170
8 am		50				150				250		190		
9 am	250	150	100				150							
10 am					150			200					100	
11 am	175	100			175				200		180			
12.00			250			100						150		130
1 pm							200			200				
2 pm	190	W		130	150			175				270		
3 pm						W			100	W	270			
4 pm								W						
5 pm	300	200				150	200			150		W		W
6 pm				190	200									
7 pm		75		W				150			100		180	
8 pm					100				200	175				
9 pm	150	100											120	
10 pm				150					175		190			175
11 pm							100		100					
12.00				50		W	100				100			
1 am													100	
2 am		W								W		W		120
3 am						120								
4 am														
5 am			150											
Waking	6 am		7.45 am		7.30 am		7.00 am		6.30 am		7.45 am		7.40 am	
Retiring	12.30 am		11.30 pm		12.51 am		Midnight		Midnight		12.30 am		11.30 pm	
Pad usage	3		1		2		4		3		5		2	

Table 3.2   *The bladder diary.* Recording volume and time of each void, fluid intake, pad usage and incontinence episodes (W). Patients also record waking/retiring time to allow calculation of nocturia.

also asked to record the time he or she is awake and asleep, which allows the accurate calculation of the urinary output at night. Patients must be instructed to continue their normal activities during the assessment to obtain an accurate representation of their normal lower urinary tract function. The ICS has recommended that voiding diaries are performed for at least 3 days. Most patients find them acceptable for use over short periods.

Frequent findings

- Normal frequency and voided volumes.
- Increased frequency and normal volumes – therefore an increased 24-hour production of urine, suggesting a high fluid intake. This may be related to diabetes mellitus or diabetes insipidus but is more usually habitual, especially with the increasing popularity of high-fluid diets.
- Reduced volumes with minimal variation in the volume voided – suggesting a bladder wall pathology such as bladder pain syndrome/painful bladder syndrome/interstitial cystitis or carcinoma in situ. (Note: An anatomical capacity measured under general anaesthesia will confirm the presence of a reduced bladder capacity due to anatomical reasons such as fibrosis or a contracted bladder. A reduced anatomical capacity often implies a low likelihood of response to conservative therapeutic modalities.)
- Reduced volumes with variation in the volume voided – suggestive of underlying detrusor overactivity as the bladder contracts at variable degrees of distension before maximum capacity, erroneously informing the patient that the bladder is full, thus resulting in urinary frequency and low and variable voided volumes.
- Increased nocturnal production of urine (nocturnal polyuria) – suggestive of cardiac failure, dependent fluid shifts in the supine position, hormonal fluid balance abnormality or idiopathic in origin. This is not necessarily a result of a urological condition.

Voiding diaries must not be overinterpreted but should be used in combination with other forms of urodynamic and urological assessment (Table 3.3).

Bladder retraining

In addition to having diagnostic benefit, voiding diaries have therapeutic value and can provide important information that is helpful in treating bladder dysfunction. This information is particularly useful for providing biofeedback during bladder retraining drills commonly used in patients with small volume frequency and urgency incontinence. Voiding diaries also

Urodynamic parameters measured by voiding diaries

Parameter	Definition
Daytime frequency	Number of voids recorded in waking hours
Nocturia	Number of voids recorded during sleep hours, with each void preceded and followed by sleep
24-h frequency	Total number of awake and sleep voids during a specified 24-h period
24-h production	Total volume of urine voided during a specified 24-h period
Polyuria	Voiding of more than 2.8 L in 24 h
Nocturnal urine volume	Total volume of urine voided during sleep hours, excluding the last void before sleeping but including the first void on waking
Nocturnal polyuria	An increased proportion of the 24-h urine output that is produced at night ($>20\%$ in young patients and $>33\%$ in more elderly patients)
Maximum voided volume (replaces the term *functional volume*)	The largest volume voided during a single micturition Particularly important when deciding how much to fill the bladder during pressure/flow urodynamics to prevent overfilling
Pad usage	Number of pads used during a specified period
Frequency of incontinence episodes	Number of incontinence episodes during a specified period
Frequency of urgency episodes	Number of urgency episodes during a specified period
Fluid intake	Volume of fluid ingested during a specified period

Table 3.3   *Urodynamic parameters measured by voiding diaries.*

often provide important feedback to the practitioner and patient so that they can objectively evaluate the effectiveness of any therapy.

CLINICAL NOTES

Example of a bladder retraining programme

To bring your bladder problem under control, you must reeducate your bladder and learn to resist early false sensations of bladder fullness. Retraining (or 'stretching') your bladder will help control leakage, and you can do this by trying to hold on for as long as possible before passing urine.

- It is important that you **do not** restrict your fluid intake.
- When you get the feeling that you need to pass urine, **suppress the urge until the sensation lessens or subsides**.
- At first this will be difficult, but as you persevere it will become easier.

Continued

25

- Sitting on a hard seat may help you hold on to your urine longer. Helpful distractors include taking deep breaths and counting backwards from 100.
- Contracting the pelvic floor muscles (Kegel manoeuvre) can also help abort the desire to void.
- If you wake up at night, try to hold on if you can; if possible, turn over and go back to sleep.
- If you have been prescribed tablets to help you pass your urine less frequently, take them regularly as directed.
- You should aim to reduce the frequency with which you pass urine to five or six times in 24 hours.

Remember:
You are trying to reeducate your bladder so that it will hold more urine. Although you may find this difficult at first, with practice it will get easier.

Example of a bladder drill
Patients are instructed to:
- hold on to their urine for a fixed time, such as an hour
- use the bladder retraining programme to suppress early urges
- gradually increase the time interval (i.e. an additional 15 minutes weekly) between voids until an acceptable voiding pattern is achieved.

PAD TESTING

Pad testing is a simple, noninvasive and objective method for detecting and quantifying urinary incontinence. It is easy to perform and interpret and provides a great deal of useful information.

Indications and aims

The principal aim is to determine the amount of urine leaked during a specified period (e.g. 1 hour), thus quantifying the severity of incontinence to both clinician and patient, as frequently the degree of incontinence is unclear from the history. In addition, the test is particularly useful to confirm the presence of incontinence when other tests (e.g. pressure/flow urodynamics) have failed to demonstrate any urinary leakage.

Method and standardization

To obtain a representative result, especially for those who have variable or intermittent urinary incontinence, the test period should be as long as possible in circumstances that approximate those of everyday life, yet it must be practical. The pad test should be conducted in a standardized fashion, and the ICS has provided guidelines on performing a '1-hour pad test'.

URODYNAMICS IN PRACTICE: 1-HOUR PAD TEST

The International Continence Society has suggested the following guidelines:

- The test should occupy a 1-hour period during which a series of standard activities are carried out.
- The test can be extended by further 1-hour periods if the result of the first 1-hour test is not considered to be representative by either the patient or the investigator; alternatively, the test can be repeated after filling the bladder to a defined volume.
- The total amount of urine leaked during the test period is determined by weighing a collecting device such as a nappy, absorbent pad or condom appliance (ensure that the collecting device has adequate capacity).
- A nappy or pad should be worn inside waterproof underpants or should have a waterproof backing.
- Immediately before the test begins, the collecting device is weighed to the nearest gram.

Typical test schedule

- The test is started without the patient voiding.
- A preweighed collecting device (pad) is put on and the first 1-hour test period begins.
- The patient drinks 500 mL of sodium-free liquid within a short period (maximum 15 minutes), then sits or rests.
- The patient walks for 30 minutes, including stair climbing equivalent to one flight up and down.
- For the remaining period, the patient performs the following activities: standing up from sitting 10 times; coughing vigorously 10 times; running on the spot for 1 minute; bending to pick up a small object from the floor 5 times; washing hands in running water for 1 minute.
- At the end of the 1-hour test, the collecting device is removed and weighed. The change of weight of the collecting device is recorded. A change of less than 1 g is within experimental error, and the patient should be regarded as essentially dry.
- If the test is regarded as representative, the subject voids and the volume is recorded; otherwise, the test is repeated preferably without voiding.
- If the collecting device becomes saturated or filled during the test, it should be removed and weighed, then replaced by a fresh device.
- The activity programme may be modified according to the patient's physical ability.

Practical points

- The total weight of urine lost during the test period is taken to be equal to the gain in weight of the collecting device(s). An increase in weight of the pad of less than 1 g in 1 hour is not considered to be a sign of incontinence, as a small weight change may be due to weighing errors, sweating or vaginal discharge.
- The test should not be performed during a menstrual period.
- A negative result should be interpreted with caution; the test may need to be repeated or supplemented with a more prolonged test.
- Any variations from the usual test schedule should be recorded so that the same schedule can be used on subsequent occasions.
- In principle, patients should not void during the test period. If they experience urgency, they should be persuaded to postpone voiding and to perform as many of the activities listed for the last 15 to 30 minutes of the test as possible to detect leakage.
- Before voiding, the collection device is removed for weighing. Patients may influence the test result by voiding prior to removing and weighing the pad.
- If voiding cannot be postponed, the test is terminated. The voided volume and duration of the test should be recorded. The results for patients who are unable to complete the test may require separate analysis, or the test may be repeated after rehydration.

Urodynamic parameters measured by pad testing

Pad testing determines the volume of leakage during a specified period. Note that 1 g is equal to 1 mL, and therefore an increase in weight of the collection device (pad) by 10 g, for example, is equal to urinary incontinence of 10 mL.

Normal values

The hourly pad weight increase in continent women varies from 0.0 to 2.1 g/hour, averaging 0.26 g/hour. With the 1-hour ICS pad test, the upper limit (99% confidence limit) has been found to be 1.4 g/hour.

URODYNAMICS IN PRACTICE: VARIATIONS TO THE PAD TEST

- Colouration of the urine with oral pyridium before pad testing can help differentiate between vaginal discharge and urinary incontinence.
- Additional changes and weighing of the collecting device can give information about the timing of urine loss.
- The collecting device may be an electronic recording pad so that the timing is recorded directly.

- Home pad tests lasting 24 to 48 hours are superior to 1-hour tests in detecting urinary incontinence; however, they are less practical and more cumbersome. The pads must be stored in an airtight container before and after use to prevent evaporation, until they have been weighed. The normal upper limit for a 24-hour test is 8 g.
- Experts who routinely perform pad testing do so for several reasons:
  - Severe patients with high volume incontinence may experience lower cure rates with antiincontinence procedures.
  - Pad testing provides an excellent objective outcome measure.

UROFLOWMETRY

Uroflowmetry is the simplest and often most useful investigation in the assessment of patients with predominantly voiding symptoms.

Indications and aims

Uroflowmetry is a noninvasive and inexpensive test that gives a great deal of information regarding voiding function by measuring the rate of flow of voided urine:

- It can often be used to support the diagnosis of bladder outflow obstruction (BOO) or detrusor underactivity, suspected from the history.
- It is an excellent screening tool for BOO, particularly when combined with measurement of residual urine volume, and is frequently the first-line screening investigation for most patients with suspected voiding dysfunction.
- It is useful for identifying those patients who require more extensive urodynamic evaluation.

Uroflowmetry is an adequate investigation for uncomplicated BOO in greater than 60% of patients. More detailed investigations are only indicated in limited situations, such as when the findings are at variance with the symptoms, if there are significant storage symptoms or if initial treatment has been unsuccessful.

Method and standardization

Uroflowmetry is performed using a flowmeter, a device that measures the quantity of fluid (volume or mass) voided per unit time (Fig. 3.1). The measurement is expressed in millilitres per second (mL/s). Patients are instructed to void normally, either sitting or standing, with a comfortably full bladder and should be provided with as much privacy as possible and comfortable

29

Fig. 3.1 *Flowmeter. Photograph of a typical flowmeter which is usually placed below a large funnel for the patient to void into. The funnel is normally placed under a commode for females; men can void directly into the funnel whilst standing. The flowmeter is usually connected to a printer device to allow graphical and numerical representation of the results. The photograph also shows results printersterm.*

surroundings to remove the inhibitory effects of the test environment. Uroflowmetry can be carried out either by itself or in combination with other techniques, such as the measurement of postvoid residual (PVR) urine. The patient should be asked if the void was representative of his or her usual voiding. (It is important that the flowmeter is regularly calibrated per the manufacturer's instructions to maintain the accuracy of the readings.)

URODYNAMICS IN PRACTICE: TYPES OF FLOWMETER

- **Rotating disk flowmeter:** The voided fluid is directed onto a rotating disk, and the amount landing on the disk produces a proportionate increase in its inertia. The power required to keep the disk rotating at a constant rate is measured, thus allowing calculation of the flow rate of fluid landing on the disk.
- **Electronic dipstick flowmeter:** A dipstick is mounted in a collecting chamber. As urine accumulates, the electrical capacitance of the dipstick changes, allowing calculation of the rate of fluid accumulation and hence the flow rate.
- **Gravimetric flowmeter:** The weight of collected fluid or the hydrostatic pressure at the base of a collecting cylinder is measured. The change in weight or pressure allows calculation of the flow rate.

Normal values

Males younger than 40 years generally have maximum flow rates greater than 25 mL/s. Flow rates decrease with age, and men older than 60 years with no BOO and a normally functioning detrusor usually have maximum flow rates greater than 15 mL/s.

Females have higher flow rates than males, usually of the order of 5 to 10 mL/s more for a given bladder volume. Exaggerated maximum flow rates are typical in women who have stress incontinence, where the outlet resistance is minimal, and in patients who have marked detrusor overactivity – the so-called fast bladder.

Interpretation

Uroflowmetry is invaluable in the assessment of voiding function for a wide range of urological conditions. Reliance should be placed on the observed flow pattern as well as on any absolute values obtained (Figs 3.2 and 3.3). The results must always be interpreted within the context of the clinical situation, recognizing the limitations of the study.

The measured flow rate is dependent on several factors, including:
- strength of detrusor contraction (detrusor contractility)
- presence of BOO
- adequacy of relaxation of the sphincter mechanisms
- patency of the urethra
- compensatory mechanisms such as abdominal straining.

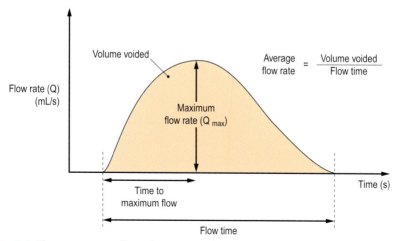

Fig. 3.2 *Flow rate recording.* *The International Continence Society nomenclature is shown. (Reproduced with permission from Tadic SD, Holstege G, Griffiths DJ. The CNS and bladder dysfunction. Neurourology and Urodynamics. 1988;7:403–426.)*

31

Fig. 3.3 Intermittent void. *The relationship between flow time and voiding time in an intermittent voiding pattern is shown.*

The flow rate and pattern give important clues to the underlying dysfunction; however, the major limitation of uroflowmetry is that the flow rate is a composite of both the function of the detrusor and the function of the bladder outlet/urethra. It is therefore impossible to determine from a flow rate alone if voiding dysfunction is due to a detrusor pathology or urethral pathology or from a combination of problems; only pressure/flow urodynamics can differentiate between such conditions. For example, prolonged flow time with an abnormally low Q_{max} may be due to bladder outflow/urethral obstruction or a poorly contractile detrusor muscle (detrusor underactivity). However, several characteristic uroflowmetry patterns have been described, and whilst these may not be specific, they give an acceptable indication of the most likely pathology in the majority of patients and allow empirical therapy to be instigated (Table 3.4).

Characteristic flow patterns

Normal – An easily distensible bladder outlet with a normal detrusor contraction results in a smooth bell-shaped curve with a rapid rise to a high amplitude peak (Q_{max}). The time to Q_{max} should not exceed one-third of the flow time. Any other patterns (flat, multiple peaks, asymmetric, prolonged) indicate abnormal voiding (Fig. 3.4a).

Fast bladder – This is an exaggeration of the normal curve and may be due to a raised end fill bladder pressure associated with detrusor overactivity or may be due to a significant decrease in outflow resistance, as can occur with stress urinary incontinence (Fig. 3.4b).

Urodynamic parameters measured by uroflowmetry

Parameter	Definition	Notes
Voided volume	Total volume expelled via the urethra	
Maximum flow rate (Q_{max})	Maximum measured flow rate	The flow curve should be assessed visually, and the Q_{max} must not be taken at the peak of an artefact but at the peak of the line of best fit for the curve.
Average flow rate	Voided volume divided by flow time	Calculation of average flow rate is only meaningful if flow is continuous and without terminal dribbling.
Flow time	Time over which measurable flow actually occurs (i.e. excluding interruptions)	The flow pattern must be described when flow time and average flow rate are measured.
Voiding time	Total duration of micturition (i.e. including interruptions)	When voiding is completed without interruption, voiding time is equal to flow time.
Time to maximum flow	Elapsed time from onset of flow to maximum flow rate	

Table 3.4 *Urodynamic parameters measured by uroflowmetry.*

Prolonged flow – This is a flow with a prolonged time to reach a low maximum amplitude and an extended flow time; often it is an asymmetric curve with a prolonged declining terminal end. This is frequently seen with BOO, although a similar pattern may be seen with a poorly contractile detrusor muscle (Fig. 3.4c).

Intermittent flow – This irregular spiking pattern is frequently due to abdominal straining to overcome the poor flow associated with BOO or a poorly contractile detrusor, although more complex outlet conditions such as sporadic sphincter activity may also cause an intermittent pattern (Fig. 3.4d).

Flat plateau – A low maximum flow rate, which plateaus for a prolonged time in a 'box-like' fashion, is characteristic of a constrictive obstruction from a urethral stricture. A urethral stricture in the presence of a normally functioning bladder usually does not cause voiding symptoms until the urethral calibre is reduced below 11 French (Fr) (Fig. 3.4e).

33

Fig. 3.4 *Characteristic flow patterns.* *(**a**) Normal – there is rapid change before and after the peak flow. (**b**) Fast bladder – an exaggeration of normal associated with high pre-micturition pressure and seen in cases of detrusor overactivity. (**c**) Prolonged flow – associated with outflow obstruction. (**d**) Intermittent flow – resulting from abdominal straining to compensate for poor detrusor contractility; a similar picture may be seen with urethral overactivity (detrusor sphincter dyssynergia or dysfunctional voiding). (**e**) Classic pattern of a urethral stricture with a long plateau.*

To provide more detailed information, a simple flow rate can be combined with a measurement of the PVR volume. If there is doubt about the diagnosis after uroflowmetry, more complex urodynamic (usually pressure/flow) studies may be required. For instance, it may be ill advised to perform a prostatectomy in men with LUTS who have a normal flow pattern, a fast bladder, or very intermittent flow and a high PVR without first determining pressure/flow urodynamics.

Practical points

There are several important factors to consider when interpreting flow rates, including:

- Volume voided – low voided volumes of less than 150 mL can lead to erroneous results and should be repeated, whereas high voided volumes of greater than 400 to 600 mL may lower flow rates by overstretching the bladder, resulting in detrusor overdistension and decompensation. (Note: Many patients complain of slower flow rates at night and during the first morning void, when the bladder is relatively overstretched.)
- The nature of the fluid – flowmeters need to be calibrated for the type of fluid being voided due to differences in specific gravity.
- Age and sex – these may alter the flow rates.
- Pattern – particularly whether the flow is continuous or intermittent.
- Position of the patient when voiding – should be noted (e.g. sitting, standing, supine).
- Free flow – a 'free flow' occurs after natural filling of the bladder, whereas a 'non–free flow' void occurs when the bladder is filled using a catheter. The free flow void is more physiological.

CLINICAL NOTES

A normal flow rate does not exclude the presence of bladder outflow obstruction (BOO)

Frequently, uroflowmetry is performed to detect the presence and severity of BOO. However, particularly in the early stages of obstruction, there may be a compensatory increase in the voiding pressure generated by the detrusor muscle, thus overcoming the obstruction. Uroflowmetry may therefore be normal in the presence of BOO. Pressure/flow urodynamics can detect BOO in such a situation. This high-pressure, normal flow voiding (>15 mL/s) occurs in approximately 7–15% of patients with BOO.

A Q_{max} less than 12 mL/s is generally considered abnormal in men older than 60 years; data suggest that approximately 90% of men with lower urinary tract symptoms and a Q_{max} less than 10 mL/s are obstructed on pressure/flow studies.

Artefacts The maximum flow rate recorded by the uroflowmetry machine is frequently misleading. Common artefacts are shown in Fig. 3.5 and include:

- Straining, causing an artificial rise in the maximum flow rate.
- Irregularities in the measured flow rate due to collecting funnel artefacts and variations in direction of the urinary stream. For example, this occurs when a man voiding into a funnel changes the point he is 'aiming' at within the funnel – so-called cruising.

Due to the kinetics of smooth muscle contraction, the detrusor is unable to generate short-lived changes in amplitude (spikes). Therefore these artefacts need to be removed by the clinician by examining the pattern and 'smoothing' the curve with a line of best fit to determine the actual Q_{max}. *It is incorrect to blindly assume that the electronically reported Q_{max} is accurate.*

It must also be remembered that any alteration in the urinary stream after the urine leaves the meatus may alter the flow and introduce artefacts. The funnel/collecting device will invariably cause such modifications. There is also a lag in the flowmeter registering the flow from when the urine left the meatus; this is unimportant in free flow uroflowmetry but is a consideration when uroflowmetry is combined with pressure/flow urodynamics (see Chapter 4).

The pattern of the flow is also altered by the speed of the recording, and the ICS has recommended that:

- 1 mL should equal 1 second on the x-axis
- 1 mL should equal 10 mL on the y-axis.

POSTVOID RESIDUAL DETERMINATION

Uroflowmetry is frequently combined with simple PVR estimation using a handheld ultrasonic 'bladder scanner' to estimate the completeness of bladder emptying. When more information on bladder anatomy and function is needed, an ultrasound cystodynamogram (USCD) can be obtained (see the next section).

An elevated PVR may represent obstruction or more commonly is a surrogate marker for detrusor underactivity, which may be due to several causes, including chronic BOO, neurogenic bladder or myogenic failure. An elevated PVR is an indication for pressure/flow urodynamics.

There are several clinical implications of an elevated PVR:

- may be an indication for prostatectomy in obstructed male patients
- requires long-term surveillance in those managed conservatively
- may be associated with hydronephrosis

Fig. 3.5 Artefacts. (**a**) The artefact (a spurious maximum flow rate of 19 mL/s) results from squeezing the prepuce of the penis during voiding. (**b**) It is eliminated, revealing a true maximum flow rate of 7.4 mL/s when the patient stops squeezing the penis. (**c** and **d**) Both flow curves show artefactual spikes, but an experienced urologist has corrected the traces (dashed line) so that the true maximum flow rates are 17.5 and 9.2 mL/s, as shown. Frequently, an artefactual spike occurs at the start of the recorded flow due to the initial flow of urine registering on the flowmeter or during the flow pattern due to abdominal straining.

- predisposes the patient to recurrent urinary tract infections and bladder calculi
- potential risk factor for acute urinary retention.

ULTRASOUND CYSTODYNAMOGRAM

The USCD combines ultrasound examination of the bladder with uroflowmetry to provide more detailed information on bladder structure and function than uroflowmetry alone.

Indications and aims

Additional information obtained during a USCD includes the structure of the bladder (shape, presence of diverticula), distal ureteric anatomy (presence of hydroureteronephrosis), completeness of bladder emptying and prostate size (Fig. 3.6).

A USCD is particularly valuable for assessing patients who may have a raised PVR (e.g. patients with suspected outflow obstruction or a poorly functioning detrusor, or if there is suspected compromised voiding after a repair procedure for stress incontinence).

The addition of ultrasound assessment is easy, requiring little specialized equipment and is noninvasive with no ionizing radiation, yet it provides a more thorough assessment of the lower urinary tract.

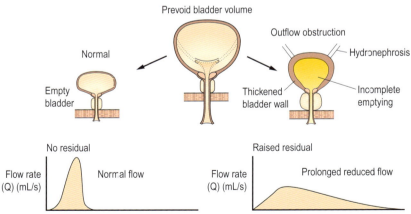

Fig. 3.6 Ultrasound cystodynamogram. *The additional ultrasonic data on the right show incomplete emptying, thickened bladder wall and bilateral hydronephrosis associated with chronic poor voiding.*

38

Method and standardization

Ensure that the patient has a subjectively full bladder before carrying out the study to provide a representative result.

URODYNAMICS IN PRACTICE: ULTRASOUND CYSTODYNAMOGRAM

- The full bladder (>200 mL) is scanned using any form of ultrasound probe allowing adequate visualization of the bladder – patients should be scanned when they feel 'full', thus providing an idea of the 'functional' bladder capacity.
- The following are noted:
  - ○ bladder wall thickness
  - ○ bladder volume
  - ○ presence of diverticulae
  - ○ distal ureteric anatomy
  - ○ prostatic volume
  - ○ presence of intravesical pathology (carcinoma or calculi).
- The patient voids into a flowmeter in private.
- A postvoiding scan is taken as soon after voiding as possible to provide accurate assessment of the true bladder postvoid residual volume.
- Interpretation of the flow rate takes account of the artefacts and factors mentioned in the uroflowmetry section of this chapter.

INTRAVENOUS URODYNAMOGRAM

The intravenous urodynamogram (IVUD) combines a conventional intravenous urogram (IVU) with uroflowmetry, thus providing markedly more information than either investigation alone.

Indications and aims

The IVUD test is of value in patients who are to undergo imaging of the upper urinary tracts using an IVU. The addition of uroflowmetry also provides a comprehensive assessment of the lower urinary tract, including an estimation of the prevoid bladder volume and the PVR. It is particularly valuable because it can be easily integrated into the routine of the radiology department and involves little additional equipment or staff training.

Method and standardization

Ensure that the patient has a subjectively full bladder before carrying out the study to provide a representative result.

URODYNAMICS IN PRACTICE: INTRAVENOUS URODYNAMOGRAM

- An intravenous urogram is obtained to assess the upper tracts.
- When the patient feels that his or her bladder is naturally full (an event that can be hastened by using a suitable diuretic), uroflowmetry is performed.
- The subsequent post-micturition film after natural micturition allows accurate assessment of the patient's true bladder residual volume.

URETHRAL PRESSURE MEASUREMENT

Originally, urethral pressure measurement and particularly urethral pressure profilometry (UPP) enjoyed a disproportionate amount of attention. However, the techniques for the investigation of urethral sphincteric function are far from satisfactory, and their clinical utility has been questioned. Therefore most experts consider them as research tools and not suitable for widespread clinical usage.

New developments in technology such as air-charged technology with true circumferential recording and ease of recording are leading to a resurgence of interest in urethral pressure measurements and may lead to an increasing understanding of the clinical utility of these tests and the clinical significance of the results. However, at present it must be concluded that these techniques remain research tools, and the various techniques need to be standardized before urethral pressure measurements can be recommended in routine practice.

The main concerns with urethral pressure measurements are as follows:

- The results obtained are extremely susceptible to experimental artefacts and the patient's degree of relaxation.
- The studies can be distressingly uncomfortable for patients, especially males.
- The mere act of measuring urethral pressures alters the intraurethral pressure and introduces artefacts.
- At rest the urethra is closed, and therefore the urethral pressure and urethral closure pressure are idealized concepts that represent the ability of the urethra to prevent leakage.
- Several techniques have been developed which do not always yield consistent values. Not only do the values differ with the method of measurement, but there is often lack of consistency within a single technique.
- The techniques as yet cannot definitively differentiate intrinsic sphincteric deficiency (ISD) from other disorders (see Chapter 5).
- The techniques as yet cannot establish the severity of the condition.

- The techniques as yet cannot provide a reliable indicator of surgical success and return to normal function following successful therapy.
- Total profile length is not generally regarded as a useful parameter in UPP.
- The information gained from urethral pressure measurements in the storage phase is of limited value in the assessment of voiding disorders, and the voiding UPP is not yet fully developed as a technique.

A detailed discussion of the various techniques is outside the scope of this book; however, a summary of the techniques is provided in the following.

Methods

Point pressure measurement

The intraluminal pressure within the urethra may be measured at a single point over a period of time:
1. **at rest**, with the bladder at a certain volume (storage phase)
2. **during stress** (e.g. coughing/Valsalva)
3. **during voiding** (voiding phase).

Urethral pressure profilometry

The intraluminal pressure can also be measured along the length of the entire urethra to produce a urethral pressure profile (UPP). This is performed by withdrawing the measuring catheter mechanically at a constant speed (Fig. 3.7). The resulting profile indicates the pressures within the urethra from the bladder neck to the meatus. Several techniques have been described, including:
- **Resting urethral pressure profile**, with the bladder at rest (storage phase). A low maximum urethral closure pressure (MUCP) on this test may be associated with ISD which may in turn be associated with a poor outcome with certain stress incontinence procedures. The test may also be useful in diagnosing sphincter damage and determining if implantation of an artificial urinary sphincter is appropriate. A high MUCP is associated with Fowler's syndrome in young women with voiding dysfunction and in patients with pelvic pain syndrome.
- **Stress urethral pressure profile**, with increased abdominal pressure (e.g. coughing/Valsalva). In stress incontinence the abdominal pressure transmission, which is thought to keep the normal urethra closed during stress, is inadequate, and therefore the urethral closure pressure decreases on increased intraabdominal pressure.

41

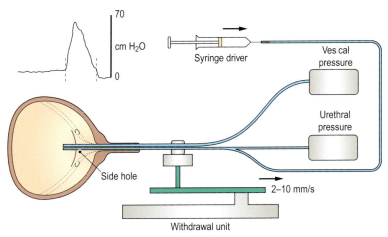

Fig. 3.7 *Urethral pressure profilometry using the perfusion method.*

- **Voiding urethral pressure profile** (voiding phase). This technique can be used to determine the pressure and site of urethral obstruction. Accurate interpretation depends on simultaneous measurement of intravesical pressure and measurement of pressure at a precisely localized point in the urethra; this localization may be achieved by a radio-opaque marker on the catheter allowing the pressure measurements to be related to a visualized point in the urethra. Pressures measured whilst voiding are the fluid pressures in the urethra and not the urethral pressure.

Fluid bridge test

A related but different test of bladder neck competence has been described. The test can detect the entry of fluid into the proximal urethra because a continuity of fluid (fluid bridge) between the bladder and urethra occurs in such a situation. The pressure transmission is measured down the infusion channel of a standard Brown–Wickham perfusion catheter (see the following) but with the perfusion switched off.

URODYNAMICS IN PRACTICE: URETHRAL PRESSURE MEASUREMENT TECHNIQUES

Perfusion method

- The perfusion method first described by Brown and Wickham is most widely used and is the measurement of the pressure needed to perfuse a catheter at a constant rate (see Fig. 3.7).

- The catheter has a dual lumen: one for pressure measurements opening at the end of the catheter and the other for perfusion via two opposing side holes 5 cm from the tip of the catheter.
- The catheter is constantly perfused at a set rate using a syringe pump (2–10 mL/min) whilst being withdrawn at a speed of less than 0.7 mL/s.

Catheter-mounted (microtip) transducers

- These eliminate errors associated with the use of fluid (leaks and air bubbles) but introduce artefacts related to the orientation of the catheter-mounted transducers on the catheter. In addition, they do not measure the urethral pressure directly but instead measure the stress imparted by the urethral tissue on the surface of the transducer only.

Balloon catheter profilometry

- This uses a small soft balloon mounted on a catheter.
- Pressure is transmitted by a fluid column to the external pressure transducer.
- It measures urethral pressure accurately, but this technique is the most difficult to use and requires frequent recalibration.

Air-charged technology (see **Chapter 4**)

- This uses a small balloon mounted on a catheter.
- Pressure is transmitted by an air column to the external pressure transducer.
- It measures urethral pressure accurately and easily, and is omnidirectional.

Practical points

When measuring urethral pressures, all systems should be zeroed to atmospheric pressure; the reference point should be taken as the superior edge of the symphysis pubis for external transducers or the transducer itself for catheter-mounted transducers. Intravesical pressure should be simultaneously measured to exclude a detrusor contraction, and subtraction of the intravesical pressure from the urethral pressure produces the urethral closure pressure profile.

The following information is essential when reporting and interpreting the results of urethral pressure studies:
- bladder fullness
- position of the patient, as posture affects the urethral muscle tone
- measurement technique
- size and type of catheter
- rate of infusion (perfusion method)
- infusion medium (liquid or gas)

- stationary, continuous or intermittent withdrawal of catheter
- rate of withdrawal
- orientation of the sensor (catheter transducers)
- period of time of recording
- manoeuvres (e.g. cough and Valsalva).

Urodynamic parameters measured by urethral pressure profilometry

TERMINOLOGY: URETHRAL PRESSURE PROFILES (Fig. 3.8)

Urethral pressure: the fluid pressure needed to just open a closed urethra

Urethral pressure profile: a graph indicating the intraluminal pressure along the length of the urethra

Urethral closure pressure profile: derived by the subtraction of intravesical pressure from urethral pressure

Maximum urethral pressure: the maximum pressure of the measured profile

Maximum urethral closure pressure (MUCP): the maximum difference between the urethral pressure and the intravesical pressure. (Note: It is thought that a low MUCP [<20 cm H_2O] may be associated with intrinsic sphincter deficiency, whereas a high MUCP may suggest bladder neck hypermobility. However, the literature on this subject is contradictory, reflecting both the variability in techniques used and inconsistency of results.)

Functional profile length: the length of the urethra along which the urethral pressure exceeds intravesical pressure

Pressure 'transmission' ratio: the increment in urethral pressure on stress as a percentage of the simultaneously recorded increment in intravesical pressure (Fig. 3.9).

NEUROPHYSIOLOGICAL INVESTIGATION

As with urethral pressure measurements, neurophysiological urodynamic investigations have failed to achieve widespread clinical usage. Neurophysiological testing allows the researcher to develop a greater understanding of lower urinary tract function, but it is uncertain what added value such testing provides to a clinician. A particular concern is that these tests tend to only be abnormal in the presence of a clinically detectable neurological condition; therefore there is very little additional new information provided by such testing that cannot be obtained by conventional pressure/flow urodynamics and a thorough neurological assessment.

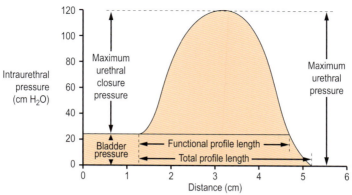

Fig. 3.8 *Diagram of a female urethral pressure profile in the storage phase.* *The nomenclature recommended by the International Continence Society is shown. (Reproduced with permission from Tadic SD, Holstege G, Griffiths DJ. The CNS and bladder dysfunction. Neurourology and Urodynamics. 1988;7:403–426.)*

Methods

Several different neurophysiological methods have been described, including:

- **Electromyography** – used to study the electrical potentials generated by the depolarization of muscle (Fig. 3.10). The action potentials can be detected by either needle electrodes placed into the muscle mass or by surface electrodes. The results are usually displayed on an oscilloscope screen, and this procedure can be done either solitarily or as part of a urodynamic investigation. Potential sampling sites include the intrinsic striated muscle of the urethra, the periurethral striated muscle, bulbocavernosus muscle, external anal sphincter and pubococcygeus muscle. Normal motor units have a characteristic waveform which can be altered by disease. In addition, during normal voiding there should be no sphincter activity. Increased sphincter activity during voiding in association with increased detrusor pressures and flow changes is characteristic of detrusor sphincter dyssynergia (see Chapters 6 and 9). This form of neurophysiological testing may also be of utility in detecting Fowler's syndrome in young females with voiding dysfunction who have been found to display peculiar sphincter activity during voiding.
- **Nerve conduction latency studies** – used to determine the time taken for a response (latency) to occur in a muscle following stimulation of a peripheral nerve.

Fig. 3.9 Pressure transmission ratio. (a) Urethral pressure profiles in a normal female at rest (left) and whilst coughing (right). During coughing, there is transmission of intraabdominal pressure (represented by the bladder trace) to the urethra in all except the distal portion of the profile. (b) Urethral pressure profiles in a patient who has urodynamic stress incontinence at rest (left) and whilst coughing (right). At rest, the bladder pressure trace is flattened compared to normal; during coughing, there is a lack of the normal transmission of intraabdominal pressure to the urethra, resulting in negative deflections in the urethral closure pressure trace. This abnormal response results from a prolapse of the urethra within a cystourethrocoele. (Reproduced with permission from Abrams P, Feneley R, and Torrens M. Urodynamics. Berlin: Springer; 1983.)

Fig. 3.10 *Muscle action potential from a urethral sphincter electromyogram.*

- **Reflex latencies** – similar to nerve conduction studies but instead assess the latency response of reflex arcs which are composed of both an afferent and efferent limb and a synaptic region within the central nervous system (CNS). This is performed by stimulation of a sensory field and recording the reflex muscle contraction. The reflex latency expresses the nerve conduction velocity in both limbs of the reflex arc and the integrity of the CNS synapse. A prolonged reflex latency therefore may be due to slowed conduction in any of these components of the reflex arc.
- **Sensory testing** – sensory function in the lower urinary tract can also be assessed by semiobjective tests that rely on the measurement of urethral or vesical sensory thresholds to a standard applied stimulus such as a known electrical current. The vesical/urethral sensory thresholds are the least current that consistently produces a sensation perceived by the subject during stimulation at the site under investigation.

UPPER URINARY TRACT URODYNAMICS

The upper urinary tract is a highly distensible system that is normally protected from the intermittent high pressure generated by the bladder by the competent vesico-ureteric junction (VUJ).

The following occur in the upper tracts under normal circumstances:
- Urine accumulates in the renal pelvis at a resting pressure of less than 5 cm H_2O.
- The pelvic pressure rises to 10 cm H_2O on distension.

47

- Urine enters the ureter to be transported as a bolus to the bladder by ureteric peristalsis at intrabolus pressures of 20 to 60 cm H_2O. Efficient peristalsis is dependent on apposition of the ureteric walls. Ureteric dilatation (whether obstructive or not) and disorders of ureteric wall mobility interfere with this process.

The normal response of the upper urinary tract to obstruction at or above the VUJ is to increase the rate of ureteric and pelvic peristalsis; however, if the obstruction remains unresolved, ureteric dilatation may occur.

Ureteric dilatation causes uncoordinated peristalsis and inefficient urine transport. As flow is reduced down the ureter, pressure rises are transmitted:

- first to the renal collecting ducts
- then along the renal tubules to the glomeruli.

If there is no parallel increase in the glomerular hydrostatic pressure, filtration will eventually decrease and renal function will become impaired.

The Whitaker test

The Whitaker test is an upper tract urodynamic study combined with antegrade pyelography (Fig. 3.11). The principal indication for the investigation is to determine if upper urinary tract obstruction exists, as a dilated upper tract neither confirms nor excludes obstruction.

The principle of the test is to perfuse the upper tract with a constant flow of contrast in an antegrade manner whilst simultaneously measuring renal pelvic and intravesical pressures. The test will differentiate patients with continuing obstruction from those with upper tract dilatation secondary to permanent alterations in the musculature/tissues of the upper tract. It may also be of utility in evaluating patients with questionable pelviureteric or VUJ obstruction or those with primary defects of the ureteric musculature (e.g. prune belly syndrome).

URODYNAMICS IN PRACTICE: THE WHITAKER TEST

- The test is performed under local anaesthesia following premedication with diazepam unless the patient has an indwelling nephrostomy catheter.
- Bladder pressure is measured via a urethral catheter connected to a transducer.
- Renal pelvic pressure can be measured through a nephrostomy tube or through a needle placed in the collecting system at antegrade pyelography – the puncture

technique must be good, because any leak from the collecting system degrades the information provided by pressure studies.

- Dilute contrast is infused through one arm of a Y connector at an initial rate of 10 mL/min, whereas the other arm of the Y is connected to a pressure transducer recording renal pelvic pressure in response to perfusion (see Fig. 3.11) – perfusion at 10 mL/min is considerably in excess of physiological rates and should stress the upper urinary tract. However, at this high flow rate the normal renal pelvis and ureters will tolerate this flow easily with minimal rise in pressure.
- Bladder pressure is continuously recorded and the subtracted pressure (pelvic pressure – bladder pressure) is automatically calculated – appropriate equipment is available in any department performing lower urinary tract urodynamics.
- Simultaneous fluoroscopy defines the anatomy of the upper tract, and spot films can be taken.

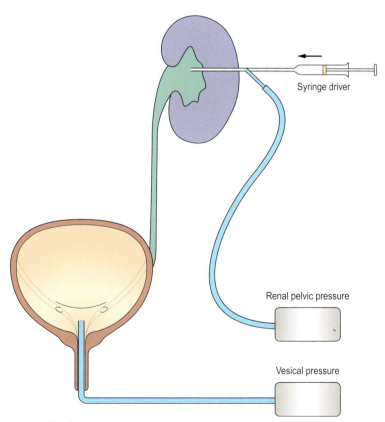

Syringe driver

Renal pelvic pressure

Vesical pressure

Fig. 3.11 Whitaker test. *The method of determining upper tract urodynamics is shown.*

Practical points

Upper urinary tract urodynamics is an invasive procedure because a percutaneous nephrostomy tract is required, and thus it should be reserved for cases where other investigations such as excretory urography and isotope renography have produced equivocal results. The main value of the Whitaker test is in providing an accurate objective assessment of obstruction to renal drainage. Significant rises in pressure are indicative of obstruction, whereas free drainage of contrast at low pressure excludes obstruction.

Using this technique, a pressure difference between the upper and lower urinary tract:

- of less than 15 cm H_2O excludes obstruction.
- of more than 22 cm H_2O confirms obstruction.
- of between 15 and 22 cm H_2O lies in the equivocal range.
- that increases equally together, then vesicoureteric reflux has occurred.

An additional indication is in patients with urinary diversion (e.g. an ileal loop). Loin pain can occur because of the high pressures generated by bowel peristalsis causing reflux up the reimplanted ureters; the extent of this can be easily assessed by upper urinary tract urodynamics.

CHAPTER 4

Pressure/flow cystometry

INTRODUCTION

In the previous chapter, several urodynamic techniques were introduced, including commonly performed and important techniques such as voiding diaries, uroflowmetry and pad testing. However, the term *urodynamics* is usually (incorrectly) used to solely describe the technique of pressure/flow cystometry.

In this chapter, pressure/flow cystometry techniques will be discussed in detail. Emphasis will be placed on correctly setting up the equipment according to International Continence Society (ICS) guidelines, correct terminology, indications for performing the procedures and how to interpret the results. Subsequent chapters discuss common lower urinary tract disorders and associated urodynamic findings in greater detail.

AIMS OF PRESSURE/FLOW CYSTOMETRY

Cystometry is necessary for equivocal or more complex cases; the principal advantage of pressure/flow studies over other urodynamic techniques such as uroflowmetry is that the simultaneous measurement of bladder pressure and voiding function allows the site of dysfunction to be localized specifically to either the bladder or the bladder outlet/urethra. In addition, cystometry provides much useful information regarding the function of the lower urinary tract during both the storage and voiding phases of the bladder cycle and in many instances can provide a definitive pathophysiological diagnosis for the lower urinary tract symptoms (LUTS) experienced.

The principal aim is to reproduce the patient's symptoms and to correlate the symptoms with the underlying urodynamic findings. This should allow a specific urodynamic question to be answered, which include:
- diagnosis
- disease severity
- most significant abnormality

- future management options
- potential postoperative problems
- results of treatment
- future problems (surveillance) in at-risk groups such as patients with neurological dysfunction.

In addition, during cystometry it is possible to define the behaviour of the bladder during both the storage and voiding phases. In the normal situation the bladder fully relaxes during storage and contracts forcefully during voiding. Likewise, it should be possible to define the behaviour of the urethra during both phases. Potential combinations of bladder and urethral function are reviewed in Table 4.1.

Pressure/flow studies also help characterize:

- bladder compliance
- bladder sensation
- bladder capacity
- flow rate (with the additional pressure data not available during uroflowmetry alone).

Pressure/flow cystometry techniques

Several different techniques have been developed to allow the synchronous measurement of bladder pressures and flow rates.

Simple cystometry – In simple cystometry, only the intravesical (total bladder) pressure is measured. This technique is not accurate, as it assumes that the detrusor pressure approximates to the intravesical pressure. A significant proportion of the pressure measured in the bladder emanates from intraabdominal structures and not from the detrusor muscle itself, since the bladder is subject to changes in intraabdominal pressure, as are all intraabdominal organs. This technique may therefore lead to an inaccurate diagnosis and is rarely performed.

Subtraction cystometry – Subtraction cystometry involves measurement of both the intravesical and intraabdominal pressures simultaneously. Real-time electronic subtraction of the intraabdominal pressure from the intravesical pressure enables the detrusor pressure component of the intravesical pressure to be isolated and analysed. During this technique the bladder is artificially filled with fluid to simulate the storage phase. This method allows the accurate determination of detrusor pressure and does not involve any radiation. It is used in urodynamic units worldwide.

Possible detrusor and urethral activity during storage and voiding

	Storage phase					Voiding phase				
	Detrusor		Urethra			Detrusor		Urethra		
	Underactive	Active	Underactive	Active		Underactive	Active	Underactive	Active	
	Normal	Abnormal	Abnormal (incompetent)	Normal		Abnormal	Normal	Normal	Abnormal (obstructive)	
	Bladder relaxation to allow filling	Detrusor overactivity, often associated with overactive bladder symptoms and urgency incontinence	Associated with stress incontinence	Maintains continence		Hypocontractile or acontractile bladder, associated with chronic detrusor muscle damage or abnormal neurology	Contraction allows forceful expulsion of urine	Opening of the urethra allows voiding with minimal resistance from the urethra	Overactive urethral sphincter may be associated with abnormal neurology; prostatic bladder outflow obstruction (BOO) increases outlet resistance	

Table 4.1 *Possible detrusor and urethral activity during storage and voiding.*

Videocystometrography (also known as videocystometry and video urodynamics) – By combining subtraction cystometry with contrast media bladder filling and radiological screening, it is possible to visualize the lower urinary tract during the storage and voiding phases. This results in the gold standard for urodynamic investigation (Fig. 4.1).

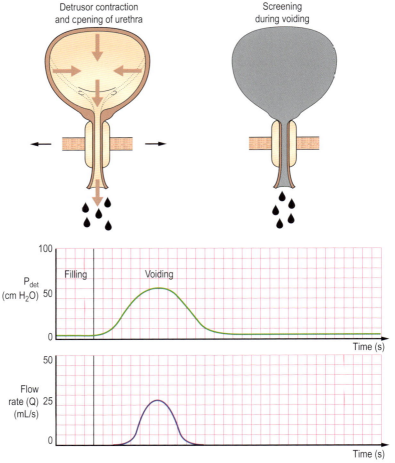

Fig. 4.1 *Normal videocystometrogram during voiding. The intraabdominal and intravesical pressures are excluded from this trace. The top left schematic shows the detrusor muscle contracting during voiding and the bladder outlet opening. The top right schematic shows the appearance during voiding of the bladder and urethra using radiological screening.*

54

Radiological screening provides valuable additional anatomical information on:
- the bladder and the urethra
- the presence of vesicoureteric reflux
- the level of any bladder outflow or urethral obstruction in the lower urinary tract
- the degree of support to the bladder base and the mobility of the urethra.

This information and the accompanying pressure/flow traces can be recorded, allowing subsequent review and discussion.

Ambulatory urodynamics (AUM) – AUM is a highly specialized form of subtraction cystometry, which contrary to other pressure/flow cystometry techniques allows the bladder to fill naturally via the kidneys and is performed over a greater length of time. AUM will be discussed further at the end of this chapter.

Risks of pressure/flow studies

The decision to perform an invasive procedure must balance the possible benefits versus the possible risks, and these must be explained to the patient when obtaining informed consent for the procedure. Risks include:
- discomfort during the procedure
- transient discomfort and dysuria following the procedure
- transient bleeding following the procedure
- urinary tract infection occurs in 2% to 4% of patients – those at high risk of infection should receive prophylactic antibiotics
- radiation exposure during video urodynamics – pregnancy must be excluded in women of childbearing age
- failure – occasionally the urodynamic question is unanswered by the study. This may be due to a failure to reproduce the symptoms, inadequate interpretation or poor technique.

Subtraction cystometry or video urodynamics?

Many urodynamic units do not have the benefit of combined fluoroscopic screening, and most patients can be adequately investigated using subtraction cystometry, particularly in the assessment of suspected detrusor overactivity (DO). Suspected stress urinary incontinence is better assessed with video urodynamics; however, it can still be evaluated during subtraction cystometry, albeit without radiological visualization of the leakage or an assessment of bladder base support and urethral mobility. Urethral pressure profilometry (see Chapter 3) and leak point pressure measurements may provide additional information in stress incontinence when video urodynamics is not available, but their use is not standardized and remains controversial. Suspected bladder outflow obstruction (BOO) can also be diagnosed during subtraction cystometry, but the addition of screening allows the level of the obstruction to be determined.

Video urodynamics provides a combined anatomical and functional assessment of the lower urinary tract and is essential for:

- investigation of complex cases in which equivocal results have been obtained from simpler investigations or previous subtraction cystometry
- investigation of patients with known or suspected neurological dysfunction (see Chapter 9)
- situations where there has been an apparent failure of a previous operative procedure.

Terminology of pressure/flow cystometry

Some general terminology related to pressure measurements is provided in Table 4.2 for reference, and additional terminology is included in the remainder of this chapter.

EQUIPMENT SETUP

The success of any pressure/flow study relies on meticulous equipment setup and adherence to strict quality control throughout the procedure. The ICS has recommended the use of fluid-filled lines and external pressure transducers during cystometry; however, if other equipment is to be used, then the principles of ensuring accurate pressure measurements specific to that equipment must still be adhered to. In addition, it is important that all equipment, including transducers, pumps and flowmeters, are regularly calibrated per the manufacturer's specific guidelines for the equipment.

A typical subtraction cystometry assessment that uses fluid-filled lines requires the following components (Fig. 4.2):

- transducers to measure pressures
- fluid-filled catheters to transmit the intravesical and intraabdominal pressures to the transducers
- a second intravesical catheter to fill the bladder with fluid (or a dual-lumen intravesical catheter $\leq$8 French (Fr))
- an infusion pump connected to the filling line, which usually works via the peristaltic principle
- a flowmeter to measure the flow rate

Terminology relating to pressure/flow cystometry		
Terminology	**Definition or urodynamic meaning**	**Notes**
Zero pressure	Should be the surrounding atmospheric pressure	Pressure recorded when the transducer is open to the environment
Reference height (level)	The level at which the transducers should be placed so that all urodynamic pressures have the same hydrostatic component	Taken at the upper edge of the symphysis pubis
Transducer	A device which converts pressure changes into an electrical signal	May be external to the patient or internally placed
Pressure	Force per unit area	Usually measured as centimetres of H_2O during urodynamics
Dampening	A specific type of artefact	Due to poor transmission of pressure to the transducer
Intravesical pressure	The pressure within the bladder	Abbreviated as P_{ves}
Intraabdominal pressure	The pressure surrounding the bladder; usually measured in the rectum but can also be measured in other sites such as the upper vagina or existing stoma	Abbreviated as P_{abd}
Detrusor pressure	The component of intravesical pressure created by forces in the bladder wall (the detrusor muscle) and calculated by subtracting intraabdominal pressure from intravesical pressure	Abbreviated as P_{det} ($P_{det} = P_{ves} - P_{abd}$)

Table 4.2 *Terminology relating to pressure/flow cystometry.*

- a computer station with appropriate connections to control the pump infusion rate that should also record the measured pressures and flow rate, as well as calculate the subtracted 'detrusor' pressure to measure the postvoid residual (PVR).

It is essential that both the urodynamicist and the person setting up the equipment and preparing the patient (if different) are familiar with the setup and are able to troubleshoot the commonly encountered problems that may occur during the procedure.

Measuring the pressures

Catheter placement

Intravesical – During cystometry the total bladder (intravesical) pressure is measured by inserting a catheter into the bladder. The catheter is usually

57

Fig. 4.2 Typical pressure flow workstation. *The workstation comprises transducers on an adjustable-height stand (**a**); a pump for bladder filling (**b**); a display, in this case with a superimposed screening image (**c**); and a uroflowmeter for use during the voiding phase of the study (**d**).*

passed via the urethra using lubricant or anaesthetic gel. In certain circumstances the catheter can be inserted via the suprapubic route. It should be ensured that the catheter is fixed securely and is in no danger of falling out. If taped to the skin, the fixation should be as near to the meatus as possible; in men, there should be no obstruction to the urethra on the undersurface of the penis.

Intraabdominal – The intraabdominal pressure is also measured so that the detrusor pressure can be accurately calculated. The measured intravesical pressure is composed of two components: the pressure created by the detrusor muscle and the pressure transmitted to the bladder from the external intraabdominal pressure. By subtracting the intraabdominal pressure from the intravesical pressure, the pressure generated intrinsically within the bladder (i.e. from the detrusor muscle) is isolated. The detrusor pressure itself is of greatest interest to the urodynamicist. The intraabdominal pressure is usually measured by inserting a catheter into the rectum; however, insertion into the upper vagina or into a preexisting stoma is also possible.

The catheter usually has a flaccid, air-free balloon on the rectal end. The purpose of the balloon is to maintain a small fluid volume at the catheter opening and to avoid faecal blockage. The balloon should only be filled to 10% to 20% of its unstretched capacity, and overfilling is a common mistake causing misleading measurements; often a slit is cut in the balloon to prevent overfilling and a tamponade effect. The rectal catheter should be inserted 10 cm above the anal verge using lubricant and taped securely, as close to the anal verge as possible.

Transducers

Three types of transducer systems are in common usage.

External fluid-charged pressure transducers – The ICS currently recommends the use of external fluid pressure transducers due to their accuracy and inherent characteristics allowing easier use with regards to zero pressure and reference height (Fig. 4.3). Urodynamics was originally developed using water-filled systems, and standardization has therefore developed from an understanding of the characteristics of fluid-filled systems. The transducers are fixed externally and are connected via fluid-filled lines to the pressure-recording catheters. Fluid transmits the measured pressures directly to the external transducer, and any interruption to the transmission of pressure waves may lead to artefacts. Common artefacts include an air bubble anywhere in the tubing between the tip of the catheter and the transducer; air is

Fig. 4.3 *External fluid transducers.* *The image at left shows a disposable casing, often referred to as the 'dome', which is attached to the fluid containing tubing. The image at right shows the transducer without a dome.*

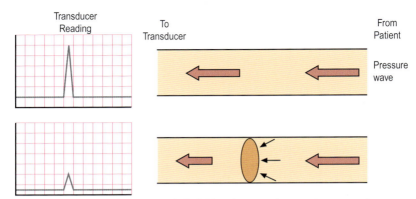

Fig. 4.4 Dampening due to an air bubble. *The upper diagram shows normal pressure transmission. The lower trace shows an air bubble being compressed and therefore 'absorbing' some of the pressure wave, leading to reduced transmission and a lower baseline and lower deflection on the trace.*

compressible, unlike fluid, and therefore a transmitted pressure wave will preferentially compress the air prior to reaching the transducer. The use of some of the pressure in compressing the air will result in a lesser wave being transmitted to the transducer, resulting in 'dampening' of the trace (Fig. 4.4). This is a common problem, and even a miniscule air bubble can cause detectable dampening in the highly sensitive transducers. It can usually be rectified by flushing the air bubble out of the system. A fluid leak or a kink in the tubing will also have similar consequences, so it should be ensured that the system is watertight during the setup procedure and that there are no kinks anywhere along the tubing. Pressure sensing is point sensitive and therefore essentially unidirectional within the fluid-filled system, albeit the pressure measurements are not so dependent on the orientation of the catheter within the bladder.

Catheter-mounted transducers – These transducers are mounted on the end of special (microtip) catheters. They do not require a fluid-filled system, and the external proximal end of the catheter is connected directly to the electronic recording system, thus making them simpler to set up than fluid-filled systems (Fig. 4.5). A reference height does not need to be set up for these systems, and they are not affected by movement artefacts. They are therefore advantageous in certain situations such as AUM, but they are not recommended by the ICS for conventional cystometry. The main disadvantage of this system is that the pressure readings are directional, depending on which way the transducer is facing or what the transducer is lying against. Furthermore, catheter-mounted transducers require regular calibration, require meticulous

Fig. 4.5 (a) Microtip (solid-state) catheter. A dual intravesical and urethral measuring microtip catheter with a transducer visible distally and a urethral transducer visible a few centimetres more proximal are shown. **(b) Transducers on a microtip (solid-state) catheter.** A closeup is shown of the distal end of a rectal microtip catheter (top) and an intravesical microtip catheter (bottom), with arrows designating the transducers.

61

cleaning and are expensive. Reference height, unlike in external fluid catheters, is at the level of the internal transducer (see later discussion). These catheters should be presoaked prior to use to allow a small amount of water absorption into the coating on the sensing area. Cleaning/disinfecting using a liquid-based method immediately prior to use is sufficient presoaking. If not cleaned by a fluid method immediately prior to use, then approximately 20 minutes of presoaking is required if the catheter is used regularly; if the catheter has not be used for some weeks, then presoaking for longer than 1 hour is required.

Air-charged pressure sensing technology – This is the newest transducer system. The system consists of reusable cables with built-in transducers and disposable catheters with a tiny balloon affixed on the distal end of the catheter (Fig. 4.6). After the disposable catheter is inserted into the patient and connected to the permanent cable, the transducer is used to 'charge' the catheter by injecting a microvolume of air into the catheter balloon. This creates a closed pressure-sensing system for accurate in vivo recording of bladder, abdominal and urethral pressures. This system is gaining popularity due to its simpler and quicker setup than fluid-charged systems. In addition, pressure sensing is not unidirectional, and the catheters are disposable, unlike with microtip catheters. The pressure measurement using the pressure sensing balloons is truly circumferential using this system, unlike fluid-filled and microtip systems, and therefore may be of particular benefit when measuring urethral pressures, as the total pressure generated by the cylindrical urethral wall is measured. In addition, these transducers are easily zeroed; similarly to microtip catheters, the reference height does not need to be set externally but is taken at the point of the internal balloon. Dampening due to a change in the transmission medium (as occurs when an air bubble is trapped in a fluid-filled

Fig. 4.6 *Air-charged pressure sensing technology.* A disposable air-charged catheter with an integral balloon attached to the permanent cable with built-in transducer is shown.

system) is not a problem in air-charged pressure sensing catheters. The pressure measurements are also not influenced by any movements of the catheter, thus decreasing artefacts; this characteristic is ideal for AUM. However, this technique does need to be further studied before it can replace fluid-filled catheters as the standard technique, and trials are currently ongoing.

Filling the bladder

In addition to intravesical pressure measuring, the bladder also requires filling with fluid during pressure/flow cystometry (Fig. 4.7).

Catheter types

Dual lumen – These are recommended by the ICS, as one dual-lumen catheter can be used for both the intravesical pressure measurement and for bladder filling (Fig. 4.8). The thinnest possible catheter should be used to limit artefacts during voiding due to obstruction of the urethral lumen. However, if the calibre of the catheter is too small, it may lead to excessive dampening of the pressure transmission and may also limit the pump rate.

Fig. 4.7 *Schematic diagram of video urodynamics.* *The bladder is filled at a predetermined rate with a radio-opaque contrast medium, with the simultaneous measurement of intravesical pressure and intraabdominal pressure. The subtracted detrusor pressure is calculated automatically, and flow is recorded with the flowmeter. This information with accompanying radiographic pictures and a sound track can be recorded, allowing subsequent review and analysis.*

Fig. 4.8 *A dual-lumen intravesical catheter.* This is used for both pressure measurement (blue channel) and bladder filling (transparent channel) with a single catheter.

The smallest currently available size is 6 Fr; however, such a small size is thought to limit the pump rate. In view of this, a slightly larger size (i.e. 8 Fr) is probably preferable.

Single lumen – If used, it requires two separate catheters to be inserted into the bladder, which is less convenient for the patient and the investigator. The filling tube can be removed during the voiding phase, but it may need to be reinserted if a second fill/void cycle is required.

A note should be made of the type, size and number of catheters utilized during an investigation.

Filling fluid

The following can all be used for filling during cystometry:
- sterile water
- normal saline
- radiological contrast – during video urodynamics.

However, it is important that the pump and flowmeter are calibrated for the fluid used, and thus it is inadvisable to change the type of filling fluid part-way through a study, as accurate calibration would not be possible.

Fluid temperature

Ideally the fluid should be at body temperature; however, it is more practical to use fluid at room temperature, and this does not appear to affect the results. Colder fluids ($<14°C$) may irritate the bladder and precipitate DO.

Quality control

Once the pressure measuring and filling apparatus are set up, it is important to ensure that the pressures are recorded correctly and any obvious issues are rectified prior to commencing the study.

Setting the zero pressure

The pressure measurements can be 'zeroed' either to the surrounding atmospheric pressure or to the internal pressure. The ICS recommends that the surrounding atmospheric pressure should be used, as it facilitates standardization of the technique and comparison of data to that from other centres.

To zero to atmospheric pressure, both the transducer measuring intravesical pressure and the transducer measuring intraabdominal pressure must be opened to the atmosphere. This is easily facilitated if three-way taps are incorporated into a fluid-filled setup (Fig. 4.9).

Fig. 4.9 Position of three-way taps in fluid-filled system. The diagram shows the position of three-way taps between the transducer and syringe and between the transducer and tubing leading to the patient. Various positions of three-way taps allow the transducer to be zeroed to atmospheric pressure, tubing to be flushed or pressure to be measured.

Setting the reference height

External fluid-filled system – The reference height is the level at which the transducers must be placed so that all urodynamic pressures have the same hydrostatic component. To ensure standardization the ICS has defined the reference height as the superior edge of the symphysis pubis. The transducers are usually mounted on an adjustable stand and should be moved so that they are level with the symphysis pubis prior to commencing the study (Fig. 4.10).

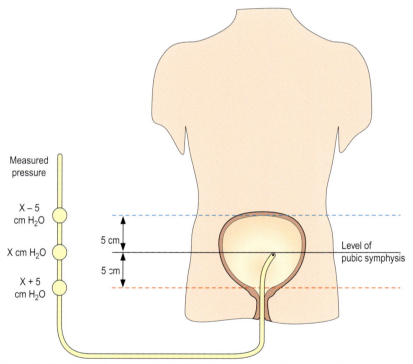

Measured
pressure

$X - 5$
cm H_2O

X cm H_2O

$X + 5$
cm H_2O

5 cm

5 cm

Level of
pubic symphysis

Fig. 4.10 *Position of external fluid-filled transducers.* *These should be set at the level of the pubic symphysis to allow standardization and comparison. Increasing the height of the external transducer lowers the measured pressure, whereas lowering the height increases the measured pressure. The position of the catheter in the organ has no effect on the measured pressure.*

URODYNAMICS IN PRACTICE: REFERENCE HEIGHT

- It is important that the reference height is kept at the level of the symphysis pubis throughout the investigation.
- Therefore any changes in patient position require the transducer height to be immediately adjusted.
- It is often difficult to maintain the transducers at the level of the symphysis pubis in fluid-filled systems when there are rapid movements, such as certain provocation tests (heel bouncing, star jumps). In addition, in fluid-filled systems, rapid movements will result in significant movement artefacts.

Microtip and air-filled systems – For microtip transducers the reference height is the transducer itself; for air-filled transducers the reference height is at the position of the internal balloon. Using these systems, it is therefore difficult to be certain of the position of the reference height or to ensure that the reference height of the intraabdominal and the intravesical lines are equal, unless screening can show the position of the catheters (Fig. 4.11). In addition, alterations in the position of the patient (i.e. supine to standing) can cause significant differences in the relative positions of the intravesical and intraabdominal transducers/balloons. In the supine position the rectal line is likely to be lower than the intravesical line, and when standing the

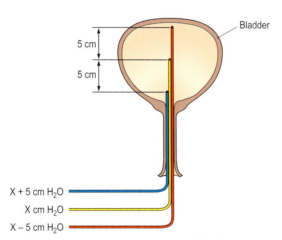

Fig. 4.11 *Position of a microtip transducer or air-filled balloon.* *The position of the internal transducer or balloon within the bladder alters the measured pressure. If the position is lower, then a higher pressure will be measured due to the extra fluid column above the transducer/balloon: a high position will therefore have a lower pressure.*

rectal line may be higher than the intravesical line. In practical terms, these differences in height are unlikely to result in a significant effect on results.

Resting pressures

Prior to commencing bladder filling, it is important to ensure that the initial values are in the expected range (Table 4.3). If the measured pressures lie outside of this range, then this suggests that a technical problem exists which needs to be rectified. Simple measures such as flushing the lines and checking for fluid leaks and kinks should be performed first.

Due to the pressure subtraction, the P_{det} should be less than 6 cm H_2O and ideally as close to zero as possible.

URODYNAMICS IN PRACTICE: TROUBLESHOOTING RESTING PRESSURES

- **If the P_{det} is too high (>6 cm H_2O)**
  - The P_{abd} may be too low – the rectal catheter may be kinked/blocked or may contain air bubbles or a fluid leak; therefore flush the system and exclude leaks and kinks.
  - The P_{ves} may be too high – the vesical catheter may have been misplaced in the urethral sphincter or the tubing may be kinked; therefore exclude kinks and, if necessary, adjust the position of the catheter.
- **If the P_{det} is negative**
  - The P_{abd} may be too high – the rectal catheter may have been misplaced, is resting against the rectal wall or the tubing may be kinked; therefore check the position and exclude kinks. The rectal balloon may have a tamponade; therefore drain a few drops of fluid from the intraabdominal measurement system or make a hole in the rectal balloon to remove excess fluid.
  - The P_{ves} may be too low – the vesical catheter may be kinked or may contain air bubbles or a fluid leak; therefore flush the system and exclude leaks and kinks.

Expected resting range of intraabdominal and intravesical pressures	
Position	**Expected range for intraabdominal and intravesical resting measurements**
Supine	5–20 cm H_2O
Sitting	15–40 cm H_2O
Standing	30–50 cm H_2O

Table 4.3 *Expected resting range of intraabdominal and intravesical pressures.*

Dampening and subtraction

Having ensured that the resting values are as expected, any dampening must be identified and rectified. This is performed by asking the patient to cough; both the intraabdominal and intravesical traces should respond equally with a rapid peak and a rapid drop, and the detrusor trace should be unaffected. A small biphasic 'blip' is normal in the detrusor trace, but any rise/fall in the detrusor pressure during the cough suggests dampening in either the intraabdominal or intravesical system (Fig. 4.12).

URODYNAMICS IN PRACTICE: ASSESS FOR DAMPENING

- Coughs to assess for dampening should be performed at the beginning and end of the investigation.
- Dampening should be assessed throughout the investigation by having the patient cough every minute (Fig. 4.13).
- Coughs should also be performed before and after any major events, such as position changes, voids and spontaneous leaks, because catheters may become displaced during these events.
- Any dampening should be immediately corrected.
- Usually the dampening is occurring in the intraabdominal or intravesical line that is deflected the least on coughing.

Fig. 4.12 Normal and dampened pressure transmission. (Left) *Good subtraction with no dampening.* **(Middle)** *Intraabdominal line dampening.* **(Right)** *Intravesical line dampening.*

69

Fig. 4.13 *Layout of a graphical display with quality control by regular coughs.*
The order of the displayed traces is shown, as recommended by the International Continence
Society. Subtraction and dampening are assessed every minute by coughs during filling and before
and after voiding.

Medications

To obtain the best indication of the unaltered underlying pathophysiology, the patient should not be taking drugs that affect LUTS. The
medications should have been discontinued sufficiently prior to the
test to allow any effects to have dissipated. We normally suggest

discontinuing 1 week prior to the study. Any variations from this ideal must be taken into account when interpreting results and should be clearly recorded.

Sometimes it is beneficial to study patients whilst taking antimuscarinic agents:

- to evaluate the competence of the outlet in a patient with mixed incontinence and whose DO is controlled with antimuscarinics
- to reassess detrusor pressure in patients with high-pressure neurogenic bladder overactivity treated with antimuscarinics.

PERFORMING PRESSURE/FLOW CYSTOMETRY OR VIDEO CYSTOMETRY

Computer display

The graphical display on the computer monitor with and without paper trace will usually have been preconfigured; however, these are modifiable and the ICS recommends for consistency that:

- the intraabdominal pressure (P_{abd}) is displayed at the top
- the intravesical pressure (P_{ves}) is displayed next
- the subtracted detrusor pressure (P_{det}) is displayed next
- the urinary flow rate (Q) is displayed at the bottom (see Fig. 4.13)
- the infused volume, voided volume, urethral pressure, electromyographic traces and video screening images are displayed optionally.

Cystometry stages

Pressure/flow cystometry is split into two phases mirroring the normal bladder cycle. The urethral and the detrusor function should be evaluated in both phases.

- Storage/filling phase (also termed *filling cystometry*):
  - commences when the pump is turned on
  - ends when the patient and the urodynamicist decide that 'permission to void' has been given (usually at maximum tolerated capacity).
- Voiding phase (also termed *voiding cystometry*):
  - commences when the patient and the urodynamicist decide that permission to void has been given or when uncontrollable voiding begins
  - ends when the patient considers that voiding has finished.

Storage phase

Having made sure that the equipment is set up correctly, is working as expected and the measurements are of good quality, then the pressure/flow cystometry can commence.

Upon starting recording:
- A cough should be performed to record the initial quality of the trace.
- The pump should be commenced at the required fill rate.
- An assessment should be made of the initial residual (see the following discussion).

Fill rate

The rate of filling should have been decided prior to beginning the procedure. The ICS originally categorized this into three fill rates:
- **slow fill:** less than 10 mL/min) – a 'physiological' filling rate, used in neurogenic patients
- **medium fill:** 10 to 100 mL/min – the most frequent filling rate
- **rapid fill:** >100 mL/min – a very rapid provocative filling rate.

In practice, most patients will be filled at a medium fill rate, and therefore the ICS has more recently decided to instead categorize fill rates as being either physiological or nonphysiological based on body weight. We would advocate a rate of 50 mL/min in nonneurogenic patients and 20 mL/min in neurogenic patients as being a good balance between performing the investigation rapidly and provoking the detrusor by an abnormally high filling rate. Quality control coughs performed every minute will therefore be every 50 mL filled in nonneurogenic patients.

Patient position

The most physiological position and the position in which most patients experience troublesome symptoms is during standing, and ideally patients should be in the standing position for some part of the filling phase of cystometry. Whilst standing, the greatest external pressure is placed on the bladder, and this may be sufficient to provoke DO. In addition, many patients only demonstrate stress urinary incontinence when standing. During the voiding phase the patient should be in the position in which he or she usually voids (commonly standing for men and sitting for women).

In practice, as the catheters are placed whilst supine, it is often helpful to commence filling in this position, as any early problems can be corrected without moving the patient back to a supine position. Following this, the patient should be brought to a standing position as soon as possible whilst the bladder capacity is being reached. However, variations in local equipment and screening facilities may require the patient to be filled in the supine or sitting positions. In addition, supine may be the only practical position for filling in certain patients, such as those with neurological dysfunction or very small children. The position should be documented throughout the test, and any changes in position will require the external transducer height to be readjusted so it remains level with the upper edge of the symphysis pubis.

Initial residual

Prior to catheterizing, the patient is asked to void as completely as possible. Following this, an assessment can be made of the residual volume at the start of the investigation. This can be performed by:

- carrying out an ultrasound bladder scan prior to catheterization
- draining the urine at the time of catheterization
- screening immediately at the start of commencing the pump (video urodynamics):
  - Allow a visual estimation of the bladder volume as the contrast diffuses with the initial residual urine to outline the size of the bladder.
- calculating the initial residual at the end using the following formula:
  - Initial residual = (volume voided + estimated volume incontinent + final residual) – volume infused.
  - The volume incontinent in practice is difficult to measure and in patients with large residuals is not usually significant.
  - The final residual is measured by draining the bladder via catheter (or by ultrasound bladder scan) at the end of the procedure.

Draining the urine at catheterization is the most direct and accurate method of determining the initial residual and attempts to ensure that the investigation commences on a completely empty bladder. However, the removal of a large volume of residual urine may alter detrusor function, especially in neurogenic patients who do not self-catheterize and in patients with hydronephrosis secondary to raised detrusor pressures, and may not represent the normal clinical situation. In these instances, the measured maximum cystometric capacity (MCC) and bladder compliance may be falsely lowered by removal of the initial residual. A similar response is seen if the bladder is filled too rapidly.

Communication

Communication with the patient is often overlooked, yet it is integral to the success of the investigation. Communication should be constant and should commence prior to catheterization with a thorough explanation of the investigation and a review of the current symptoms and recent voiding diary. The investigation is unfamiliar and embarrassing to most patients, and the entire urodynamic team must be sensitive to this and must continually ensure that the patient feels at ease. It is helpful to ascertain if any particular activities (e.g. bending, heel bouncing, hand washing) provoke the symptoms so that these can be integrated into the cystometric assessment. It is essential to relate the urodynamic findings to the patient's symptoms throughout the study, as this is vital to the interpretation of the urodynamic findings.

The patient should be asked to inhibit the desire to void or leak throughout the storage phase and should be told to immediately disclose any urgency sensations felt or any incontinent episodes during the storage phase. The patient also needs to inform the team if any suprapubic or abdominal pain occurs during filling. Usually if pain is experienced, then filling should be discontinued and the voiding phase commenced. Any events need to be recorded on the trace.

It is important that the bladder sensations associated with cystometric filling are recorded, and this requires that bladder sensations are explained fully to the patient and the patient knows to inform the urodynamicist as soon as these sensations occur (see the following discussion).

Bladder sensations

Bladder sensations are difficult to evaluate because of their subjective nature; the patient needs to inform the urodynamicist about sensations relating to fullness as soon as they occur, and these should be recorded on the trace. Good communication is required to ensure that the patient informs the urodynamicist of the sensations experienced without the urodynamicist prompting the patient to the degree that 'words are put in the patient's mouth'.

TERMINOLOGY: BLADDER SENSATIONS AS DEFINED BY THE INTERNATIONAL CONTINENCE SOCIETY

First sensation of bladder filling: When the patient first becomes aware of the bladder filling.

First desire to void: The feeling that would lead the patient to pass urine at the next convenient moment, but voiding can be delayed if necessary.

Strong desire to void: The persistent desire to void without the fear of leakage.

Maximum cystometric capacity: In patients with normal sensation, this is the volume at which the patient feels he or she can no longer delay micturition.

Urgency: A sudden compelling desire to void, which is difficult to defer.

Bladder pain: This should not occur during filling; if it occurs, the site and character should be specified.

CLINICAL NOTES: BLADDER SENSATION

The overall bladder sensation can be described as being normal, increased or reduced:
- **reduced** – diminished sensation throughout bladder filling
- **normal** – normal occurrence of bladder sensations
- **increased** – an early first sensation or an early desire to void and/or an early strong desire to void, which occurs at a low bladder volume and which persists.

Detrusor function during the storage phase

Normal detrusor function – During the storage phase the bladder should be relaxed and compliant to bladder filling with little or no change in detrusor pressure. Any detrusor activity prior to the voiding phase is therefore abnormal and termed as *involuntary detrusor activity* (IDA).

Detrusor overactivity – This is characterized by involuntary detrusor contractions (IDCs) during the storage phase. It was previously termed *detrusor instability* or *detrusor hyperreflexia* (when associated with known neurological disease). The occurrence of associated urgency should be documented on the trace. DO can be:
- spontaneous or provoked
- phasic – having a characteristic waveform of repeated waves of DO
- terminal – an IDC occurring at cystometric capacity, which cannot be suppressed and results in incontinence/voiding
- idiopathic – when there is no defined cause for the overactivity. This is commonly seen associated with the overactive bladder syndrome.
- neurogenic – when there is an underlying neurological condition causing the lower urinary tract dysfunction.

URODYNAMICS IN PRACTICE: PROVOCATION MANOEUVRES

- Provocative manoeuvres are techniques used during the storage phase to provoke detrusor overactivity.
- They should be used in patients suspected from their history to have detrusor overactivity but who have not demonstrated any involuntary detrusor contractions during the storage phase.
- They are therefore usually done towards the end of filling when the patient has reached or is nearly at his or her maximum cystometric capacity.
- Examples include bending, changing posture, coughing, jogging on the spot, running water, hand washing, heel bouncing, star jumping, increasing the filling rate and using cooled filling fluid (the latter two examples need a new fill cycle to commence).
- Often determining the most useful provocation manoeuvre follows from asking the patient what provokes his or her symptoms and attempting to recreate this during the investigation.

If DO is detected, then the volume at which the contraction occurred should be recorded, as should the rise in amplitude above the baseline (Fig. 4.14). The duration of the contraction should also be noted. It is also important to document if urgency was experienced in association with the IDC; usually a marker can be electronically placed on the trace when urgency occurs. Any associated incontinence should also be documented.

CLINICAL NOTES: TERMINAL DETRUSOR OVERACTIVITY

- Frequently, as the patient with detrusor overactivity reaches bladder capacity, he or she has an involuntary detrusor contraction (usually sustained and of high amplitude compared to previous contractions during the filling phase). Such a terminal contraction is often associated with significant urgency, and the patient often becomes increasingly uncomfortable.
- Often in this situation the patient either spontaneously voids or the urodynamicist instructs the patient to void due to the increasing discomfort, resulting in a void 'on top of' an overactive detrusor contraction.
- However, when a patient voids during a terminal contraction, it is not possible to definitively determine if:
  - the patient has high pressure voiding suggestive of BOO
  - the patient has normal voiding
  - the patient has low-pressure voluntary voiding suggestive of detrusor hypo-contractility.

- In this situation it is incorrect to interpret the voiding pressures, as patients may be misdiagnosed (e.g. erroneously diagnosed) with obstruction in addition to detrusor overactivity.
- Compounding this, if the trace is read retrospectively and it is unclear at what point the permission to void was given, then the trace can often be interpreted in a variety of ways depending on what point it is assumed that permission to void was given.
- Ideally the patient should be refilled and the voiding phase repeated prior to the patient developing a terminal contraction, thus allowing the lower urinary tract function during the voiding phase to be fully appreciated.

Fig. 4.14 Detrusor overactivity. *The volume at which detrusor overactivity commenced, the rise in amplitude and duration, the leakage on the uroflowmeter, an urgency marker and a subsequent quality control cough are all shown.*

Bladder compliance

Bladder compliance describes the intrinsic ability of the bladder to change in volume without a significant alteration in the detrusor pressure. A bladder can either be normally compliant or poorly compliant (hypocompliant).

$$\text{Compliance}\,(\text{mL/cm}\,H_2O) = \frac{\text{change in volume}\,(\Delta V)}{\text{change in detrusor pressure}\,(\Delta P_{det})}$$

Calculation of compliance requires two standard points to be chosen on the trace. The change in volume and the change in pressure are calculated between these two points, allowing the compliance between the two points to be calculated. The ICS suggests the following two standard points of measurement:

1. At the start of filling: P_{det} usually is zero, and volume (V) is usually zero.
2. At cystometric capacity or immediately before any detrusor contraction that caused significant leakage (and therefore caused the bladder volume to decrease).

The standard points should not be measured at the time of a detrusor contraction, as this would give a falsely poor compliance; instead they should be taken at the baseline detrusor pressure at that point.

CLINICAL NOTES: CHECKING BLADDER COMPLIANCE

- Normal compliance is greater than 30 to 40 mL/cm H_2O.
- Abnormal compliance is less than 30 to 40 mL/cm H_2O.
- An abnormally poor compliance is often an artefact of the unnaturally high filling rates that are used during cystometry (excluding ambulatory urodynamics).
- If compliance is seemingly poor, it is often useful to slow the fill rate:
  - If compliance improves at the slower rate, then an artefact was present and filling should continue at the slower rate (Fig. 4.15).
  - If compliance remains poor, then true hypocompliance is present.

Bladder capacity

Cystometric capacity – This is the bladder volume at the end of the storage phase when permission to void is given and the investigation moves into the voiding phase. This is usually the MCC (see the following discussion); however, if it is not the MCC, then the cystometric capacity should be further

Fig. 4.15 Bladder compliance. (**a**) Normal compliance with each 30- to 40-mL increase in bladder volume causing an increase in pressure of less than 1 cm H_2O. (**b**) Seemingly poor compliance. (**c**) Artefactual poor compliance due to high fill rate; when filling is stopped the pressure decreases, and when it is recommenced at lower rate the compliance is seen to be normal. At the end of filling, it is recommended to wait approximately 30 seconds before recording the end filling pressure. (**d**) True poor compliance: stopping filling does not cause a drop in pressure, and filling further at any fill rate continues to show poor compliance.

defined with a reason why filling was stopped (e.g. pain, large infused volume, high detrusor end filling pressure).

Maximum cystometric capacity – In patients with normal sensations, this is the volume at which the patient feels that he or she can no longer delay micturition due to a strong desire to void. Where there is altered or absent sensation, the MCC cannot be measured and the cystometric capacity should instead be recorded.

During cystometry, under normal circumstances the bladder should fill to a capacity of approximately 500 mL before there is a strong desire to void. There is probably no benefit in overfilling patients with volumes above 650 to 700 mL, as little additional information is likely to be obtained.

79

Urethral function during the storage phase

During storage the urethral closure mechanism should be fully active and competent, thereby preventing incontinence (it cannot be overactive). Clearly the urethral closure mechanism can be poorly functioning and therefore incompetent. The urethral closure mechanism is therefore described as being:

- **Normal** – maintains continence in the presence of increased intra-abdominal pressure, although it may be overcome during DO, leading to incontinence
- **Incompetent** – allows leakage in the absence of a detrusor contraction
- **Demonstrating urodynamic stress incontinence** – involuntary leakage of urine during increased intraabdominal pressure in the absence of a detrusor contraction (previously termed *genuine stress incontinence*)
- **Demonstrating urethral relaxation incontinence** – leakage due to urethral relaxation in the absence of raised intraabdominal pressure or DO.

To assess the urethral function, the patient can be asked to increase his or her intraabdominal pressure (usually by coughing or performing the Valsalva manoeuvre); on video urodynamics the leakage of contrast can be easily seen, as can any associated hypermobility of the bladder. If the patient is positioned over a flowmeter, then the leakage may be detected on the flow trace. If urethral function is normal during storage, then there should be no leakage of contrast (in the absence of a detrusor contraction).

Leak point pressures

During the storage phase, leak point pressures can also be assessed. Two leak point pressures have been defined by the ICS.

Abdominal leak point pressure (ALPP) – This is the intravesical pressure at which urine leakage occurs due to increased abdominal pressure in the absence of a detrusor contraction.

The ALPP acts as a measure of the ability of the bladder neck and the urethral sphincter mechanism to resist increases in intraabdominal pressure. It may have value in determining if intrinsic sphincter deficiency is present, which may lead to stress urinary incontinence. The terms *Valsalva leak point pressure* (VLPP) and *cough leak point pressure* (CLPP) are sometimes used to describe the methods of increasing the intraabdominal pressure. A CLPP is thought to be the most clinically relevant, but it is difficult to measure due to the rapidity of the event. A VLPP is slower and therefore easier to perform, but it is not as clinically relevant, as it is difficult to instruct patients to carry this out in a reproducible fashion.

Detrusor leak point pressure (DLPP) – This is the lowest detrusor pressure at which urine leakage occurs in the absence of either a detrusor contraction or increased intraabdominal pressure.

The DLPP is used frequently to predict upper tract dysfunction in patients with neurological conditions associated with reduced bladder compliance and poor voiding. It measures the capacity of the bladder neck and urethral sphincter mechanism to resist increased pressure. A high detrusor pressure and high DLPP may be dangerous to the upper urinary tract. Although defined as being measured in the absence of a detrusor contraction, many urodynamicists perform the DLPP during an IDC. A cutoff of 40 cm H_2O has been suggested as the threshold for concern regarding potential effects on the upper tracts but is not an absolute value, as lower pressures can also result in upper tract dysfunction.

The methods of performing ALPP and DLPP unfortunately are not standardized, and it is therefore difficult to compare results between centres and assess the clinical relevance of the findings. When recording a leak point pressure, several variables should be recorded to document the conditions under which the test was performed. These include:

- the site of pressure measurement:
  - rectal
  - vaginal
  - bladder.
- the cause of the increased pressure:
  - cough
  - Valsalva.
- the bladder capacity at the time of assessing the leak point
- the baseline pressure used for the test:
  - the true zero intravesical pressure
  - the value of P_{ves} measured at zero bladder volume
  - the value of P_{ves} measured immediately before the cough/Valsalva manoeuvre (usually at 200 or 300 mL bladder capacity)
- the presence of prolapse
- the presence of straining (contraction and relaxation of the pelvic floor)
- the method of detecting the leak (e.g. screening, artificially coloured urine [dye], changes in electrical conductance, flowmeter).

Video urodynamic screening during the storage phase

Video urodynamics is an excellent method for evaluating the urethral outlet in female patients who have urinary incontinence. When standing partially obliquely, the position of the bladder neck at rest and during increased intraabdominal pressure (coughs, Valsalva) can be seen. In addition, leakage can be directly visualized and recorded.

Frequently beaking of the bladder neck is encountered during increased intraabdominal pressure. This is probably a normal finding and is common in continent females. This should be differentiated from the rectangular-shaped incompetent bladder neck seen in intrinsic sphincter deficiency (see Chapter 5).

In the semilateral/oblique position, the bladder neck can be differentiated from a dependent cystocoele, and this position also helps in the evaluation of the size and functional significance of a cystocoele.

During storage, other abnormalities of the bladder can be visualized, including bladder diverticula, fistulae and any vesicoureteric reflux (particularly if associated with DO) (Fig. 4.16).

Voiding phase

The voiding phase of cystometry commences when the patient and the urodynamicist decide that permission to void has been given or when uncontrollable voiding begins. In practice, in patients without any neurological dysfunction, this occurs when the MCC has been reached.

During this phase the detrusor initially contracts without a change in bladder volume; this is termed *isovolumetric contraction*. Once the bladder outlet 'opens' and urine begins to be expelled, the bladder continues to contract, resulting in a decrease in the bladder volume. At the completion of voiding the detrusor relaxes and the urethra/bladder outlet 'closes'. When the patient feels that voiding has ended, this phase ends and the storage phase begins again.

During the voiding phase, via the use of a flowmeter connected to the urodynamic equipment, flow rate parameters in addition to pressure data can be obtained and correlated with each other.

Uroflowmetry parameters that can be obtained were described in Chapter 3 and include:
- flow rate (Q)
- maximum flow rate (Q_{max})
- voided volume
- voiding time
- flow time
- average flow rate
- time to maximum flow.

a

b

ci

cii

d

e

Fig. 4.16 *Anatomical pathologies discovered during video urodynamics.* (*a*) *Large bladder diverticulum.* (*b*) *Small bladder diverticulum and stress urinary incontinence.* (*c*) *Vesicoureteric reflux: mild left reflux (i) and marked bilateral reflux and hydronephrosis (ii).* (*d*) *Vesicovaginal fistula.* (*e*) *Urethral diverticulum.*

Usually during a pressure/flow study the Q_{max} and voided volume are recorded and an assessment is made of the voiding time to determine if the void is prolonged.

Pressure parameters that can be obtained during the voiding phase are applicable to the abdominal, intravesical and detrusor pressure traces (Fig. 4.17) and include:

- **Pre-micturition pressure** – the pressure recorded immediately before the initial isovolumetric contraction. The detrusor pre-micturition pressure is probably the most clinically relevant.
- **Opening pressure** – the pressure recorded at the onset of urine flow. The intravesical opening pressure is likely to be the most clinically relevant. An adjustment for flow delay must be made for this measurement to be accurate.
- **Opening time** – the time from initial rise in detrusor pressure to onset of flow; this refers to the initial isovolumetric contraction period. An adjustment for flow delay must be made for this measurement to be accurate.

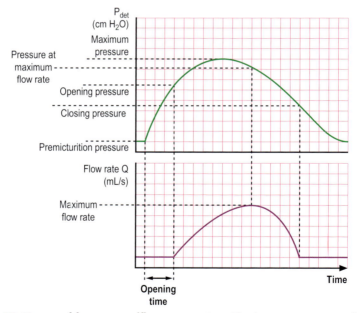

Fig. 4.17 Measurable pressure/flow parameters. *This diagram assumes that a flow rate delay adjustment has been made prior to correlating the various pressure and flow parameters.*

- **Maximum pressure** – the maximum value of the measured pressure (i.e. the peak amplitude of the voiding pressure curve). The maximum detrusor pressure (P_{det}max) is clinically relevant in determining the presence of BOO or a poorly contractile detrusor.
- **Pressure at maximum flow** – the pressure recorded at maximum measured flow rate. This is termed the $P_{det}@Q_{max}$ when referring to the detrusor pressure at maximum flow rate. This is also very helpful in determining the presence of BOO or a poorly contractile detrusor muscle. This parameter is used in calculating the BOO index (see Chapter 6) or the bladder contractility index. An adjustment for flow delay must be made for this measurement to be accurate.
- **Closing pressure** – the pressure measured at the end of measured flow. The intravesical closing pressure is likely to be the most clinically relevant. An adjustment for flow delay must be made for this measurement to be accurate.
- **Minimum voiding pressure** – the minimum pressure during measurable flow but not necessarily equal to either the opening or closing pressure.

URODYNAMICS IN PRACTICE: FLOW DELAY

- The flow delay is the time delay between a change in bladder pressure and the corresponding change in measured flow rate.
- Pressure measurements are nearly instantaneous.
- However, flow measurements encounter a delay from the time the urine leaves the urethral meatus until they are measured by the flowmeter. During this time the urine travels through the air, is collected in the collecting device and is channelled to the flowmeter where the flow rate is measured.
- This delay is variable and is dependent on the equipment being used and how it is set up.
- The delay tends to be longer in men who void whilst standing compared to women who void whilst sitting. This is due to the difference in distance from the urethral meatus to the flowmeter.
- The delay is usually between 0.5 and 1 second but can be as long as 2 seconds.
- Ideally the delay should be calculated for the equipment in use and a correction made when correlating flow rates to pressure measurements, such as when measuring the $P_{det}@Q_{max}$, opening pressure, closing pressure and opening time.
- To correct for the delay the flow rate trace should be moved to the left by an amount equal to the flow delay. The measured pressures will then correspond with the flow rates achieved by those pressures (Fig. 4.18).

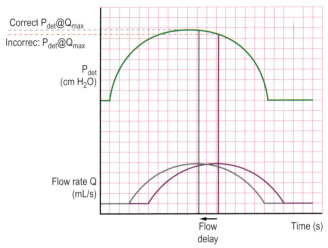

Fig. 4.18 *Flow rate delay.* The red line shows the recorded flow rate, which must be shifted to the left (blue line) by the amount of the delay, to determine the actual position of the flow trace in relation to the pressure readings.

Normal values

During voiding the patient's bladder should empty completely with a maximum detrusor pressure of 25 to 50 cm H_2O.

The maximum urinary flow rate should be:

- greater than 30 to 35 mL/s in women
- greater than 25 mL/s in men younger than 40 years
- greater than 15 mL/s in men older than 60 years.

Detrusor function during the voiding phase

Normal detrusor function – Normal voiding is achieved by a voluntary continuous detrusor contraction which leads to complete emptying of the bladder within an acceptable time span. During the voiding phase, high pressures may be encountered with BOO, because the recorded detrusor pressure is not only dependent on the magnitude of the detrusor contraction but also on the degree of outlet resistance. Therefore significant resistance, as is seen in BOO, may lead to elevated detrusor pressures. In addition, the detrusor may compensate for BOO by increasing the magnitude of contraction to expel urine through the increased resistance. Conversely, if urethral resistance is low, this may be reflected by a low-pressure contraction, which is commonly seen in male patients following prostatectomy.

Detrusor underactivity – This underactivity is defined as a contraction of reduced strength and/or duration, resulting in prolonged bladder emptying and/or a failure to achieve complete bladder emptying within a normal time span. The symptom complex that can result is termed *underactive bladder*.

Underactive bladder – An underactive bladder is characterized by a slow urinary stream, hesitancy and straining to void, with or without a feeling of incomplete bladder emptying and dribbling, sometimes with storage symptoms. Underactive bladder occurs in association with diverse pathophysiologies; based on current knowledge, there is no single distinguishing symptom. Storage symptoms are varied and may be highly prevalent, including nocturia, increased daytime frequency, reduced sensation of filling and incontinence. Underlying mechanisms of storage symptoms are diverse and often related to a significant PVR urine volume. Underactive bladder often results in a PVR volume remaining in the bladder on the completion of voiding. If during free flow uroflowmetry a PVR is not demonstrated, then any raised PVR during the urodynamic assessment can be considered as an artefact due to the artificial circumstances of the test and the presence of an in situ urethral catheter.

Acontractile detrusor – An acontractile detrusor does not demonstrate any contractile activity during urodynamic assessment. However, one must consider that some patients with a 'bashful' bladder cannot generate a detrusor contraction in the laboratory setting.

After-contraction – Occasionally a detrusor contraction which occurs immediately after micturition has ended is encountered on urodynamics. The significance of this finding is unknown, and it has been suggested that it may be associated with DO, but this is by no means always the case (Fig. 4.19).

Urethral function during the voiding phase

Normal urethral function – During the voiding phase the urethra should open and be continuously relaxed to allow the bladder to be emptied at normal intravesical pressures. The urethra can therefore not be underactive (incompetent) during voiding; however, it may be overactive due to failure to adequately and continuously relax, or it may have an anatomical obstruction such as benign prostatic enlargement or urethral stricture. Pressure/flow studies allow the degree of the overactivity/obstruction to be assessed, and with the aid of video urodynamics the precise anatomical location can be determined.

Fig. 4.19 *After-contraction.* *A large after-contraction greater than the original voiding contraction is shown on this trace.*

Bladder outflow obstruction (BOO) – This is a generic term for any obstruction seen during the voiding phase of pressure/flow studies. It is usually diagnosed by studying synchronous flow rate and detrusor pressure data and is characterized by increased detrusor pressures and reduced flow rates (see Chapter 6).

Dysfunctional voiding – This is an intermittent and/or fluctuating flow rate due to involuntary intermittent contractions of the periurethral striated muscle during voiding in neurologically normal patients.

Detrusor sphincter dyssynergia – This occurs when there is a detrusor contraction concurrent with an involuntary contraction of the urethral and/ or periurethral striated muscle. It may prevent any expulsion of urine in occasional circumstances. The condition tends to occur in patients with a suprasacral neurological lesion (see Chapters 6 and 9).

Nonrelaxing urethral sphincter obstruction – A nonrelaxing, obstructing urethra may result in reduced urine flow and tends to occur in patients with a sacral or infrasacral neurological lesion (e.g. meningomyelocoele) or radical pelvic surgery.

CLINICAL NOTES: THE STOP TEST

- During voiding in a video urodynamic study, the male patient can be asked to stop voiding.
- Normally the contrast is 'milked back' from the distal sphincter mechanism proximally through the bladder neck into the bladder.
- If there is obstruction at the level of the bladder neck, contrast will be trapped within the prostatic urethra (Fig. 4.20).
- This sudden change to an isovolumetric contraction during the stop test leads to a characteristic intravesical and detrusor pressure spike (Fig. 4.21).

a   b

Fig. 4.20 *Abnormal stop test in bladder neck obstruction.* *(a) Video urodynamic screening during voiding shows bladder neck obstruction. (b) 'Trapping' of urine within the prostatic urethra due to bladder neck obstruction when the patient voluntarily inhibits voiding is shown.*

89

Fig. 4.21 Isometric pressure contraction during a stop test. *The detrusor pressure spike during the stop test was thought to be a sign of detrusor power. This is not particularly useful or of diagnostic value.*

Video urodynamic screening during the voiding phase

Contrast screening during the voiding phase allows the bladder outlet and urethra to be assessed and is particularly useful in men with suspected BOO. The position of the obstruction can often be clearly seen, as can features such as a prostatic indentation at the base of the bladder due to an enlarged prostate. Other abnormalities such as ureteric reflux on voiding and urethral diverticula may also be discovered.

Postvoid residual urine

The PVR is the volume of fluid remaining in the bladder at the end of micturition. Its measurement forms an integral part of the pressure/flow study. However, voiding in unfamiliar surroundings can produce unrepresentative results, as may voiding on demand with a partially filled or over-filled bladder. It must be remembered that the residual volume reflects a relative impairment in detrusor function.

Important factors in the interpretation of residual volume include:
- The time interval between voiding and residual urine estimation.
- Reentry of urine into the bladder after micturition; if there is vesicoureteric reflux, then the residual urine may be falsely interpreted.
- Urine in bladder diverticula following micturition; a diverticulum can be regarded as part of the bladder or conversely can be regarded as being outside the functioning bladder when interpreting the PVR.
- An isolated finding of raised PVR requires confirmation before being considered significant.
- The residual volume can be usefully related to the functional bladder capacity estimated from a frequency/volume chart. A ratio of more than 30–40% has been arbitrarily suggested to reflect significance.

The PVR at the end of the study can be measured by draining the bladder via the intravesical catheter or by an ultrasonic bladder scan. The PVR can also be roughly estimated (with experience) by screening following voiding during video urodynamics to assess the final volume remaining in the bladder.

Completion of a pressure/flow study

On completion of the voiding phase the patient should perform a further cough to assess the subtraction quality before the recording is terminated. If there are any doubts regarding the quality of the study, the presence of artefacts or if a significant problem occurred such as the urethral or rectal catheter falling out during voiding, the study should be repeated. A nonconclusive study may also need to be repeated.

Immediately following the recording, any markers that are required should be placed on the recording. The flow rate delay should be accounted for, and any automatically generated values for urodynamic parameters in both the filling and voiding phases should be counterchecked manually. Frequently, analysis software mistakes artefacts for clinically relevant data; this counterchecking is therefore imperative to ensure accuracy, and any discrepancy should be edited. A printout of the values should be obtained along with the trace to allow for retrospective review.

It is often helpful to record the data obtained on a standard proforma, and this can be useful when interpreting the results and writing the study report (Fig. 4.22). The study report should be comprehensive and should state if the patient's symptoms were reproduced during the study. It should also answer the clinical questions that led to the test being performed, and the activity of both the bladder and urethra, where appropriate, during both the storage and the voiding phases should be stated. If more than one abnormality is discovered during the study, the most clinically significant

91

Conventional urodynamic report

Patient Details   *Date of study:*   /   /

		1	**Fill Number**	2

Filling
- Fill rate (mL/min) ☐☐☐ ☐☐☐
- Baseline P_{det} (cm H_2O) ☐☐☐ ☐☐☐
- First sensation filling (mL)* ☐☐☐ ☐☐☐
- Cystometric capacity (mL)* ☐☐☐ ☐☐☐
- Compliance (0 = normal; 1 = reduced) ☐ ☐

Overactivity
- Fill (0 = nil; 1 = phasic; 2 = nonphasic) ☐ ☐
- Cough ☐ ☐
- Posture ☐ ☐

Contraction no.	1	2	3	4	5		1	2	3	4	5
Vol. at contraction											
Max. rise in P_{det}											

Pre-micturition pressure (cm H_2O) ☐☐☐ ☐☐☐

*Filling volume (need to add initial residual in formal data recording)

Voiding
- Opening P_{det} (cm H_2O) ☐☐☐ ☐☐☐
- $P_{det.max}$ (cm H_2O) (Not $P_{det.iso}$) ☐☐☐ ☐☐☐
- P_{det} at peak flow (mL/s) ☐☐☐ ☐☐☐
- Peak flow rate (mL/s) ☐☐.☐ ☐☐.☐
- $P_{det.iso}$ (cm H_2O) ☐☐☐ ☐☐☐
- After contraction   (0 = no; 1 = yes) ☐ ☐
-                         P_{det} (cm H_2O) ☐☐☐ ☐☐☐
- Volume voided (mL) ☐☐☐ ☐☐☐
- Residual urine (mL) ☐☐☐ ☐☐☐
- Calculated initial residual urine (mL) ☐☐☐ ☐☐☐

		R	L

Video
- Bladder outline ☐   VUR Grade ☐ ☐
  - 1 = normal; 2 = trabeculated;   Grade as defined by International Reflux Study Group (Grades 1–5)
  - 3 = sacculated; 4 = multiple diverticula

	Males	Females

- Bladder neck ☐ ☐
  - In men: 1 = normal opening with void; 2 = poor opening
  - In women: 1 = closed; 2 = open with fill;
  - 3 = open with standing; 4 = open with stress

- Stop test (M)/position (F) ☐ ☐
  - In men: 1 = normal; 2 = trapping present; 3 = equivocal; 9 = not done
  - In women: 4 = well supported; 5 = descent on stress; 6 = prolapse

- Prostatic urethra ☐ 1 = normal opening; 2 = attenuated;
  - 3 = DSD; 4 = indeterminate

- Anterior urethra ☐ 1 = normal; 2 = stricture; 3 = unsure

Comments/Report

Fig. 4.22 *Example proforma used for recording results of pressure/flow cystometry.*

abnormality should be stated; this may require further discussion with the patient following the study. Finally, the study report should contain a recommendation for further investigations or treatment if appropriate.

How to interpret the trace

In addition to calculating the subtracted detrusor pressure, measurement of both the intraabdominal and the intravesical pressures allows the urodynamicist to easily determine if intravesical pressure changes emanate from within or external to the bladder by monitoring all three pressure lines. Three common patterns encountered are presented next (Fig. 4.23 and Table 4.4).

Activity external to the bladder

Intraabdominal activity occurs when the patient coughs, talks, performs Valsalva, changes position or performs any other physical activity.

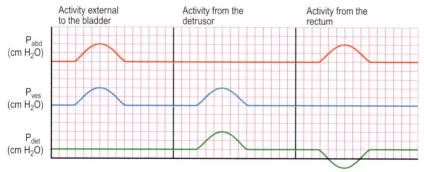

Fig. 4.23 Common trace patterns. *The diagram shows the three common patterns: activity external to the bladder (intraabdominal activity), activity emanating from the bladder (detrusor activity) and activity from the rectum.*

	Interpreting changes in pressure			
	Frequent causes	P_{abd}	P_{ves}	P_{det}
Activity external to the bladder	Cough, Valsalva, movement, talking, etc.	Raised	Raised	Unchanged
Activity emanating from the bladder	Detrusor contraction (voluntary or involuntary)	Unchanged	Raised	Raised
Rectal activity	Rectal contraction (voluntary or involuntary)	Raised	Unchanged	Lowered

Table 4.4 *Interpreting changes in pressure.*

Intraabdominal activity will cause both the intraabdominal and the intravesical pressures to rise synchronously. There should be no change in the detrusor pressure (if subtraction is adequate).

Activity emanating from the bladder

Detrusor contractions emanating from the bladder and during the filling phase, if involuntary, are a sign of DO, whilst during voluntary voiding they are uninhibited and therefore normal.

Detrusor activity will cause both the detrusor and the intravesical pressures to rise synchronously. There should be no change in the intraabdominal pressure (if subtraction is adequate).

Rectal activity

During rectal contractions the pressure in the intraabdominal trace will rise by virtue of the position of the catheter tip in the rectum. However, this pressure is not transmitted to the other intraabdominal organs, such as the bladder. Therefore the intravesical trace will be unaffected by the rectal contractions. Since during electronic subtraction the detrusor pressure is calculated by subtracting the intraabdominal pressure from the normally higher intravesical pressure, a sudden rise in only the intraabdominal (rectal) pressure causes an artefactual negative deflection of the detrusor trace which is characteristically a mirror image of the intraabdominal trace. Repeated rectal contractions can result in a detrusor trace that can easily be mistaken for phasic DO.

URODYNAMICS IN PRACTICE: INTERPRETATION TIPS

- Start by looking at the intravesical trace. If a change in pressure is seen, look at the detrusor followed by the intraabdominal trace.
- If the intravesical trace has changed synchronously with the detrusor trace, then this is genuine detrusor activity, but double check that the abdominal trace has not changed.
- If instead the intraabdominal trace has changed synchronously with the intravesical trace and there is no change in the detrusor pressure, then the activity emanates from outside the bladder and is not due to detrusor activity.
- However, if the intraabdominal pressure is a mirror image of the detrusor trace, then rectal contractions are occurring. The detrusor trace is an artefact in this case.
- With experience, interpreting these changes becomes second nature, but frequently interpretation is difficult due to multiple events occurring simultaneously (e.g. a detrusor contraction and abdominal straining).
- Interpretation is also hindered if the subtraction and quality of the recording are poor.

Troubleshooting

Artefacts are common and may lead to errors in the interpretation of results. They should be promptly detected by continually observing the trace; if an artefact is present, the study and further bladder filling should be temporarily halted. The cause of the artefact should be determined and the fault should be rectified. Prior to recommencing filling, the quality of subtraction should be reassessed with coughing.

Ensuring that the resting values are feasible

Please see the 'Resting pressures' section presented earlier in this chapter (p. 68) on ensuring that the initial resting values are feasible, and troubleshoot as suggested.

Poor subtraction and dampening

A urodynamic study may be difficult to interpret if subtraction is poor due to dampening. The line with the lowest amplitude on coughing is usually the cause of the poor subtraction and should be investigated first. Another clue to the cause of damping is the direction of the deflection of the subtracted detrusor pressure. Normally a cough should produce a small biphasic blip in the detrusor trace; however, an obviously positive deflection suggests intraabdominal line dampening, whereas an obviously negative deflection suggests intravesical line dampening (see Fig. 4.12).

If dampening in a line appears inadequate, flush the line to clear out air bubbles, ensure that there is no kinking in the line, check that all connections are secure with no fluid leakage and check the position of the line. As a last resort, replace the measurement catheter (may be blocked/defective); if no better, a transducer error (rare) should be suspected. After each attempt at remedying the problem, ask the patient to cough to determine if the subtraction has improved.

Negative rectal pressure

A negative rectal pressure adds to the total bladder pressure, and therefore the subtracted detrusor pressure may be higher than the total bladder pressure (Fig. 4.24). This is usually prevented by calibrating the lines adequately at the start of the study and avoiding air bubbles and kinks in the rectal line. In addition, when not using a special rectal balloon catheter, a finger cot should be placed around the rectal catheter to prevent blockage of the line

95

Fig. 4.24 *Pressure/flow trace obtained when a negative rectal pressure artefactually adds to the total bladder pressure.* The resulting subtracted detrusor pressure is artefactually higher than the intravesical pressure. This is seen at the start of this trace, with the negative rectal deflection curve (mimicking a detrusor contraction) and also gradually as the rectal pressure falls throughout the trace, leading to a rising detrusor pressure; this could easily be misinterpreted as poor bladder compliance. The end filling pressure should be interpreted from the intravesical pressure line in this case.

by faeculent material and a slit should be cut in the finger cot to prevent tamponade when flushing out the line. The finger cot is easily made by cutting the finger off a surgical glove and attaching this to the distal end of the rectal catheter.

Loss of trace activity

The trace should be 'active' (i.e. small second-by-second variations should be seen). If the line loses this activity and becomes a 'flat line', then there has been a total loss of pressure monitoring, possibly due to a measuring catheter falling out, a loss of pressure signal reaching the transducer due to fluid leakage, a transducer failure or a loose connection between the transducer and the monitoring computer. The line can easily be checked by asking the patient to cough or perform a Valsalva manoeuvre.

Sudden changes of pressure

Sudden large changes of pressure suggest that either the vesical or rectal catheters have moved. They may completely fall out, causing the pressure reading to dramatically drop, or they may move into an area of higher pressure, such as the vesical catheter moving from the bladder into the urethral sphincter (Fig. 4.25). Misplaced catheters should be promptly moved into the correct location. The catheters may need to be changed if they fall into a nonsterile area.

Fig. 4.25 *An uninterpretable study due to artefacts.* Prior to voiding when the patient appears to be straining, there is poor subtraction and the intravesical line appears to be malfunctioning. On commencing voiding the intravesical catheter is ejected, leading to an abrupt loss in the intravesical signal. (Reproduced with permission from WHO 4th International Consultation on Benign Prostatic Hyperplasia.)

AMBULATORY URODYNAMICS

Introduction

Conventional pressure/flow cystometry has several shortcomings, including:

- a 'nonphysiologically' high filling rate
- a short period of assessment
- being performed in a stationary position
- usually being performed in an unfamiliar environment for the patient.

It is therefore a nonphysiological assessment and may not give an accurate representation of the patient's lower urinary tract function. DO is detected using a conventional pressure/flow study in only about 50% to 60% of patients who have LUTS highly suggestive of DO. Despite the shortcomings, conventional pressure/flow studies remain the gold standard investigation of lower urinary tract dysfunction and are performed far more frequently than AUM.

AUM overcomes many of these limitations by providing a more physiological assessment of the patient's condition. During AUM, the bladder is not artificially filled but instead is filled by natural urine production from the kidneys. The test is usually done over a much longer period of time than a conventional study, ranging from a couple of hours up to 24 hours in some instances. The patient is able to perform some everyday activities, including actions which may provoke the troublesome symptoms, and the patient is free of the fixed urodynamic apparatus of conventional pressure/flow cystometry, with the monitoring taking place outside of the urodynamic laboratory.

Indications

AUM procedures are much more time consuming to perform and require regular monitoring to ensure that the catheters have not become displaced. It remains debatable as to whether they are appropriate for widespread clinical usage. To date, the technique has not been standardized and the measurement parameters not adequately defined by the ICS.

The procedure should be reserved for situations where conventional pressure/flow studies have failed to explain or reproduce the symptoms and where further knowledge of the function of the lower urinary tract is likely to aid subsequent management.

Equipment

The basic equipment needed for an AUM study comprises:

- a vesical and a rectal catheter; these tend to be catheter-mounted (micro-tip) transducers, although developments in air-charged transducers will allow AUM to be performed with these as well
- a portable storage device to record data (Fig. 4.26); this device is connected to the catheters/transducers and records the pressure readings. The device is worn by patients for the duration of the study. Developments in Bluetooth/wireless technology allow real-time monitoring of the pressures via a personal computer (PC). Most storage devices are battery powered and allow information to be collected for several hours. Extra channels on the devices may also collect measurements of urine loss and urethral pressure.
- a PC for downloading, processing and plotting the data
- a uroflowmeter which communicates the flow data to either the portable storage device or the PC used for monitoring the study.

Performing an AUM study

AUM assessments should only be performed by those experienced in performing conventional pressure/flow cystometry. Most of the principles of setting up and performing a high-quality conventional study are relevant

Fig. 4.26 *A modern Bluetooth portable ambulatory urodynamic device.* The device can be carried by the patient using a strap. The urodynamic catheters are attached to the connectors on the back of the device (just visible). The device also has event buttons for the patient to use.

during AUM studies. The transducers should be calibrated before the investigation and should be zeroed to atmospheric pressure.

Often a patient will be left unattended for a considerable length of time during an AUM study, and therefore it is imperative that the quality of the pressure recording and the subtraction be stringently assessed at the start by coughing and/or performing the Valsalva in the supine, sitting and erect positions. All catheters should be securely fixed to the patient to limit any danger of becoming displaced during movement. The urodynamicist must be convinced of the quality of measurements before proceeding with the investigation.

The quality of the measurements should be reassessed periodically during the course of a study, and the patient should be asked to cough regularly throughout and prior to terminating the monitoring and also before any voiding episodes so that on retrospective analysis the quality of the subtraction can be determined.

The procedure for performing an AUM assessment is not standardized, and therefore it is important that the method used is stated. Information to be recorded includes:

- initial residual urine
- urine leaked during study – assessed by weighing pads before and after use throughout the study or by electronic assessment of leakage (e.g. using a conductance channel to determine when leakage occurs)
- the time and volume of voids, including the flow rate, will be recorded throughout the study using a flowmeter
- length of the study
- final residual on study completion.

In addition, events should be recorded by the patient, ideally on the portable storage device, including:

- initiation of voluntary voids
- cessation of voluntary voids
- episodes of urgency
- episodes of discomfort or pain
- time and type of any specific provocative activities
- time and volume of fluid intake
- episodes of urinary leakage.

Analysis of results

The quality of the trace should be assessed by carefully checking the plausibility of the recordings and the adequacy of the subtraction. A poor-quality trace may not be suitable for quantitative analysis, although it may still yield some clinically useful information.

The storage and voiding phases should be identified during the trace, and any markers should be correlated to these. Using the same principles used during conventional pressure/flow studies, the function of both the bladder and the urethra/bladder outlet should be determined during both the storage and the voiding phases. In particular, troublesome symptoms should be correlated to the recorded findings to try to determine the pathophysiology of the symptoms.

Frequently the results following AUM are different from those obtained during conventional pressure/flow studies. In many cases, DO is not identified during conventional studies in patients strongly suspected of DO, yet IDA is picked up on the AUM study. Conversely, many patients not suspected of having DO (including asymptomatic volunteers in research studies) display IDA during AUM assessment. The significance of IDA in asymptomatic patients or IDA without associated urgency in symptomatic patients is currently unknown.

The explanation for these apparent differences between AUM and conventional urodynamics may relate to the circumstances associated with the ambulatory test. Artificial filling may be relatively insensitive, being too fast to allow detection of 'normal' or 'physiological' detrusor activity. However, although filling is natural during AUM, it is not physiologically suitable to have catheters in situ for protracted periods such as 3 to 4 hours. Voiding parameters should be more physiological during AUM, as less overfilling of the bladder should occur and the results during voiding should be more representative, despite a catheter being in situ during voiding.

Further research is needed to assess the significance of the findings during AUM and to determine the range of normality, and therefore AUM should not be used as a routine study but should be reserved only for carefully selected cases.

CHAPTER 5

Storage disorders and incontinence

INTRODUCTION

Storage disorders are common in both men and women and are often associated with urinary incontinence. Overactive bladder (OAB) syndrome affects approximately 12% of adult males and females in the population, and the prevalence increases with age, whilst urinary incontinence affects millions of individuals worldwide, 85% of whom are women. More than one-third of healthy elderly women and approximately 50% of institutionalized females suffer from incontinence, with estimates indicating that as many as one in four women experience urinary incontinence during their lifetime. Urgency and mixed urinary incontinence become proportionally more prevalent with age, whilst stress urinary incontinence (SUI) is more prevalent in middle age (Fig. 5.1)

OAB and particularly urinary incontinence carry a considerable social stigma; many sufferers are unable to continue with their daily activities, and many give up their employment. Not only are the symptoms troublesome, but they are extremely embarrassing and can have profound psychological, social, sexual and hygienic impacts. Many patients adopt elaborate coping mechanisms including voiding frequently, mapping out the location of toilets, drinking less or wearing dark clothing to mask incontinent episodes. Others resort to wearing incontinence pads or sanitary towels.

However, many successful treatments are available for these conditions, and therefore it is important that sufferers are offered a suitable treatment; frequently urodynamic studies are required to determine the most appropriate management choice. A simple algorithm for the investigation of incontinence is shown in Fig. 5.2.

OVERACTIVE BLADDER SYNDROME AND URGENCY INCONTINENCE

OAB syndrome is defined as urgency, with or without urgency incontinence, usually with frequency and nocturia. OAB can only be diagnosed if infection or other obvious pathologies that may cause the symptoms are excluded. OAB is also known as urgency syndrome and urgency/frequency syndrome. These symptom combinations are frequently associated with demonstrable detrusor overactivity (DO) during the filling phase of pressure/flow cystometry.

CLINICAL NOTES: PATIENT EVALUATION OF STORAGE DISORDERS AND INCONTINENCE

History
- Storage symptoms
- Factors that induce leakage
- Pad usage and volume leaked
- Coping mechanisms
- Obstetrical history
- Drug therapy including previous treatments
- Surgical history

Physical examination
- Palpable enlargement of the bladder postvoid residual volume
- Stress incontinence on coughing (preferably when the bladder is full)
- Pelvic organ prolapse on coughing/Valsalva
- Urethral mucosal prolapse
- Introital atrophy
- Pelvic floor muscle tone
- Abnormal neurology

Investigations
- Urinalysis
- Postvoid residual
- Pad testing
- Bladder diary

Must exclude
- Urinary tract infections
- Other significant lower urinary tract abnormalities such as bladder carcinoma or calculi (a urine sample should always be assessed for the presence of haematuria, pyuria or infection)
- Chronic retention with overflow incontinence

OAB can be further categorized as:
- OAB-dry, where there is no associated urinary incontinence
- OAB-wet, where there is associated urgency urinary incontinence.

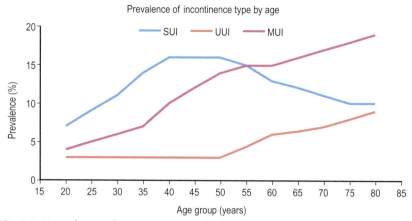

Fig. 5.1 *Prevalence of stress, urge, and mixed urinary incontinence, urge urinary incontinence by age.* *Value estimates of pooled data. SUI, Stress urinary incontinence; UUI, urge urinary incontinence; MUI, mixed urinary incontinence. (Adapted from epidemiological studies of Reynolds WS, Dmochowski RR, Penson DF. Epidemiology of stress urinary incontinence in women.* Current Urology Reports. *2011;12(5):370–376.)*

It is believed that the driving force within OAB is the symptom of *urgency*, defined as the complaint of a sudden compelling desire to pass urine, which is difficult to deter (Fig. 5.3). Urgency may compel the sufferer to void more frequently than normal and to wake from sleep to void. Increased frequency can also partly be a result of an adaptive or coping mechanism to suppress urgency. If urgency is severe and the patient has little warning or is not able to reach a toilet in time, then urgency incontinence may occur. Approximately 30% of patients with OAB have urgency incontinence, although the prevalence increases significantly in the elderly with multiple comorbidities.

Urinary urgency is commonly associated with DO. Traditionally, DO and therefore urinary urgency were hypothesized to result as a consequence of dysfunction of the efferent innervation of the bladder. However, it is likely that this relationship is more complex, as DO most probably occurs as a consequence of stimulation of afferent feedback to the limbic zone of central nervous system releasing the inhibitory control of the pontine micturition centre. Current evidence suggests that most therapy directed at the treatment of OAB acts via an improvement in the sensory symptom of urgency with a reduction in frequency, urgency incontinence and nocturia and an increase in the functional bladder capacity. Indeed, it is recognized that a significant proportion of the effect of antimuscarinics may be an action on cholinoceptors located on sensory nerves and that the action of

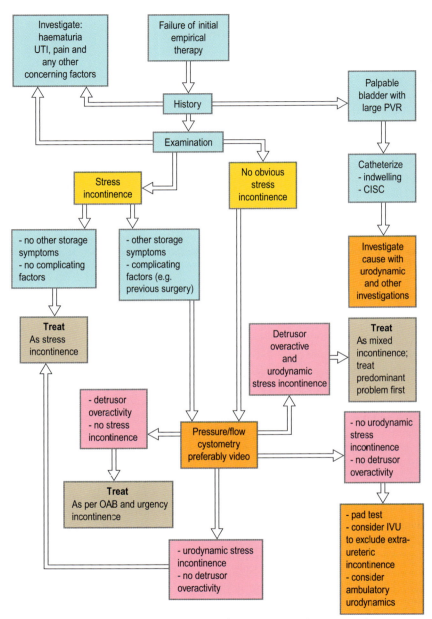

Fig. 5.2 *Algorithm for the investigation of urinary incontinence.* *Initial investigations should focus on differentiating between detrusor overactivity and urodynamic stress incontinence, although the conditions frequently coexist as mixed incontinence. CISC, Clean intermittent self-catheterization; IVU, intravenous urogram.*

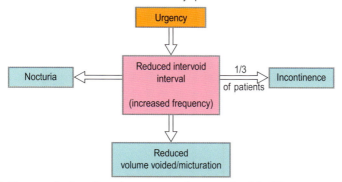

OAB syndrome: a symptomatic sequence

With static intake, urgency episodes reduce the intervoid interval and result in the other symptoms of OAB

Fig. 5.3 *Urgency is the pivotal symptom of overactive bladder.* Urgency drives the other storage symptoms.

antimuscarinics directly on detrusor muscle cholinoceptors is less important than previously believed to be the case.

Although most patients with OAB with or without urgency incontinence are described as having an 'idiopathic' problem, several other clinical causes should be considered:

- intravesical abnormalities (i.e. infection, foreign body, bladder carcinoma)
- neurogenic disease
- bladder outflow obstruction (BOO) in elderly men, urethral valves in boys, bladder neck dyssynergia in young men, pelvic floor dyssynergia and consequent on obstructing cystourethropexy
- iatrogenic (e.g. following operative treatment of stress incontinence)

Frequently the symptoms are triggered by certain events such as running water, 'key in the door', 'foot on the floor', giggling, exertion or female orgasm.

Management of overactive bladder and urgency incontinence

Many patients are treated empirically, often by their primary care physician. If successfully managed and if important pathologies such as bladder carcinoma (Fig. 5.4) and urinary tract infection have been excluded, then there is often little need for further investigations. Frequently, however, the patient may have equivocal symptoms or the condition may not respond to initial

107

a

b

Fig. 5.4 Other causes of storage symptoms. (a) Superficial transitional cell carcinoma of the bladder in a patient with predominant storage symptoms. (b) Cystoscopic evidence of a suture and bladder calculus in a patient with storage symptoms following an abdominal hysterectomy.

therapy; in such circumstances the patient should be referred to secondary care for a more detailed evaluation and a greater range of management options. Successful management of OAB requires that the condition be accurately diagnosed and differentiated from other lower urinary disorders such as stress incontinence.

Available and emerging treatment choices include:

- **Fluid intake advice** (reduce volume, reduce tea/coffee/alcohol)
- **Bladder training and bladder drill**
- **Anticholinergic (antimuscarinic) therapy:**
  - Oxybutynin (oral and transcutaneous)
  - Tolterodine (oral)
  - Trospium chloride (oral)
  - Solifenacin (oral)
  - Fesoterodine (oral)
  - Propiverine (oral)
  - Darifenacin (oral).
- **Beta-3 agonist therapy:**
  - Mirabegron (oral).
- **Synthetic vasopressin analogue** (particularly nocturia and nocturnal enuresis [NE]):
  - Desmopressin.
- **Intradetrusor botulinum toxin injections:**
  - Type A.
- **Neuromodulation:**
  - Sacral neuromodulation (mechanism unknown but may act to stimulate the Aδ myelinated fibres, especially at the S3 level; probably enhances sphincter/pelvic tone and may inhibit the detrusor reflex)
  - Paraurethral stimulation
  - Pudendal nerve stimulation
  - Posterior tibial nerve stimulation.
- **Surgery:**
  - Augmentation enterocystoplasty
  - Autoaugmentation (rarely performed)
  - Denervation (abandoned)
  - Urinary diversion:
    - ileal or colonic conduit
    - continent diversion
    - suprapubic catheter.

Note that tricyclic antidepressants such as amitriptyline are no longer recommended for use in the elderly with OAB symptoms owing to the side effects that can occur.

Urodynamics in overactive bladder and urgency incontinence

Voiding diaries – These should be used during the initial evaluation and subsequent monitoring to give an estimate of the frequency and voided volumes, including response to treatment. They are also useful to confirm the existence of nocturnal polyuria. Prior to performing invasive urodynamics, a voiding diary will give an estimate of the bladder capacity, and this information should be used to prevent overfilling during the assessment.

1-hour pad test – This test is useful in patients strongly suspected of urinary incontinence but who have failed to demonstrate any leakage on other investigations such as video urodynamic pressure/flow studies (Fig. 5.5). Approximately 30% of patients with urgency incontinence have a normal pressure/flow study. The test also gives a quantification of the degree of incontinence, as patients are usually inaccurate when asked to quantify the leakage.

Uroflowmetry – Uroflowmetry is not a particularly useful test in this condition, although it may be beneficial to exclude those with voiding dysfunction as a cause of their storage symptoms, such as men with mixed lower

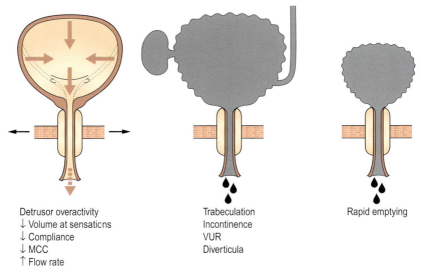

Detrusor overactivity	Trabeculation	Rapid emptying
↓ Volume at sensations	Incontinence	
↓ Compliance	VUR	
↓ MCC	Diverticula	
↑ Flow rate		

Fig. 5.5 *Possible video urodynamic findings during detrusor overactivity.* MCC, *Maximum cystometric capacity; VUR, vesicoureteric reflux.*

urinary tract symptoms (LUTS). This testing should be performed prior to pressure/flow cystometry to provide a representative indication of the voiding pattern that is likely to be encountered during invasive cystometry.

Pressure/flow cystometry – This is the gold standard test for detecting DO, which is characterized by involuntary detrusor contractions during the filling phase. DO is thought to be the underlying cause for the symptom of urgency which drives the other symptoms in OAB and which may cause urgency incontinence. Pressure/flow cystometry should be used when a patient has been refractory to empirical therapy to confirm the presence of DO before proceeding to further treatment. It is essential before considering any invasive treatment, such as botulinum toxin therapy or surgery. In addition to clarifying the diagnosis, it will help characterize other aspects of lower urinary tract function that may predict problems following an invasive procedure. For example, a patient with concurrent voiding dysfunction may be more likely to require clean intermittent self-catheterization (CISC) following botulinum toxin therapy.

Cystometry is also valuable in determining the underlying diagnosis in patients with a mixture of storage and voiding symptoms, such as men who demonstrate both DO and BOO. Similarly, in women with a mixture of symptoms suggestive of both urgency incontinence and stress incontinence, video cystometry is invaluable in determining if both conditions are present (mixed incontinence) and which is the predominant problem requiring focused treatment. Note that the presence of urgency (but not urgency incontinence) and stress incontinence is known as mixed symptoms.

Nonurodynamic tests – Several validated questionnaires are available to determine the severity of the condition and the impact on quality of life. These are useful in both the initial assessment of severity and to monitor the impact of treatment. Common questionnaires include the King's Health Questionnaire (KHQ), the Patient Perception of Bladder Condition (PPBC) questionnaire, the International Consultation on Incontinence Modular Questionnaire (ICIQ), the Overactive Bladder Questionnaire (OAB-q) and the Short Form-36 (SF-36) questionnaire.

Urodynamic findings in overactive bladder and urgency incontinence (Table 5.1)

Detrusor overactivity

The characteristic finding of DO during pressure/flow cystometry is shown in Fig. 5.6. In patients with a known neurological cause for the lower urinary tract dysfunction, this is described as neurogenic detrusor overactivity

Possible findings during urodynamic testing of patients with overactive bladder or urgency incontinence	
Voiding diaries	• Increased daytime frequency, usually >8 times daily
	• Nocturia
	• Reduced voided volumes with variable amounts
	• Urgency, if recorded
	• Incontinence associated with urgency, if present and recorded
1-Hour pad test	• >1.4-g increase in weight
Uroflowmetry	• Possible exaggerated flow rate due to high voiding pressures
Pressure/flow cystometry (see Fig. 5.5)	• Detrusor overactivity during the filling phase, often associated with urgency and incontinence
	• Reduced volumes at which first sensation, first desire and strong desire occur
	• Possible poor compliance
	• Reduced maximum cystometric capacity
	• High pre-micturition pressure
	• Fast opening time
	• High flow rate with rapid emptying
	• Time to maximum flow is reduced (often <2 s)
	• Stop test – the isometric pressure contraction is often high (>50 cm H_2O), rarely possible to perform due to the force of the detrusor contraction
	• After contraction (unknown significance)
	• Trabeculation of the bladder and occasionally diverticula during screening (video urodynamics)
	• Vesicoureteric reflux in association with high detrusor pressures (both with DO and during voiding) during video urodynamics screening (rare)

Table 5.1 *Possible findings during urodynamic testing of patients with overactive bladder or urgency incontinence.*

(NDO; see Chapter 9), whereas when the aetiology is unknown, it is described as idiopathic detrusor overactivity (IDO). DO was previously called *detrusor instability*, and NDO was previously called *detrusor hyperreflexia*.

If DO is detected, it should be ascertained if there is associated urgency and if the urgency sensation is the same as the troublesome symptom that the patient normally experiences. The volume at which DO occurs and the rise in amplitude should be documented as described in Chapter 4, as should any associated leakage. It should also be stated if the DO was spontaneous or provoked.

Frequently, phasic (systolic) contraction activity with increasingly frequent and higher amplitude contractions occurs as the bladder continues

Fig. 5.6 *High-pressure detrusor overactivity.* Note the rise in intravesical activity which is mirrored in the detrusor trace. This is the hallmark of detrusor activity, as the lack of activity in the intraabdominal trace confirms that the activity has emanated from within the bladder.

to be filled (Fig. 5.7). Often a large terminal contraction occurs, at which time the patient feels that he or she can no longer delay micturition and has therefore reached maximum cystometric capacity. The patient should be allowed to void voluntarily at this point. If voiding is delayed, the patient will frequently be incontinent (Fig. 5.8).

Increasingly forceful DO associated with urgency can cause significant discomfort for the patient, and incontinence is embarrassing. Therefore, if the presence of DO has answered the 'urodynamic question', then there is no need to significantly delay entering the voiding phase of the study, as little additional information is likely to be gained.

Cough-induced incontinence

Frequently the abrupt change in intraabdominal pressure during coughing provokes urinary incontinence (Fig. 5.9). This is often confused with stress incontinence on the history alone but during video urodynamics DO is seen immediately following a cough with associated urinary leakage. Changing patient position (i.e. to the standing position) may similarly trigger DO.

Fig. 5.7 Phasic detrusor overactivity. *A wave of detrusor contractions is shown, in this case with each contraction rising in amplitude and being of slightly longer duration.*

Involuntary contraction of the detrusor muscle during filling phase

Bladder pressure greater than urethral pressure

Leakage into urethra

Urethra relaxes and incontinence occurs

Fig. 5.8 *Mechanism of incontinence during detrusor overactivity.*

STRESS INCONTINENCE

Stress incontinence is predominantly a female problem. Depending on the definition and the population studied, the prevalence of SUI is estimated

Fig. 5.9 ***Cough-induced detrusor overactivity.*** *If this is associated with leakage, then it must be differentiated from stress urinary incontinence; in both conditions, there is leakage associated with coughing.*

to affect between 4% and 35% of the adult female population, with an apparent increase in prevalence with age. In men, stress incontinence is most commonly seen in patients following a radical prostatectomy.

The current International Continence Society definition of *stress incontinence* is 'the complaint of involuntary leakage on effort or exertion, or on sneezing or coughing'. If involuntary leakage is observed during increased abdominal pressure, in the absence of a detrusor contraction during a urodynamic assessment, then the patient is described as having *urodynamic stress incontinence*. This term replaces the older term *genuine stress incontinence*.

Stress incontinence can affect females of any age and any parity. However, it is particularly common in multiparous women who have had traumatic or prolonged vaginal deliveries and is usually associated with loss of pelvic floor support and/or damage to the sphincter mechanism. This results in either:

- descent or hypermobility of the bladder neck and proximal urethra
- intrinsic sphincter deficiency (ISD).

It is important to recognize that these two mechanisms are not dichotomous but represent a continuum on which many patients have features of both (see Chapter 2).

115

Management of stress incontinence

Initial therapy can be commenced empirically by the primary care physician. However, if this fails the patient should be evaluated in secondary care for consideration of invasive management.

Available treatment choices include:

- **Fluid intake advice**
- **Pelvic floor muscle training**
- **Devices:**
  - pads
  - adult nappies/diapers
  - cones
  - urethral plugs
  - electrical stimulation.
- **Bulking agents** (to increase urethral resistance when it is less than that of the intravesical pressure at rest)
- **Sphincter cell injection therapies** (currently at an investigative stage – therapies to regenerate the sphincteric cells in those with a relative degree of ISD)
- **Surgery:**
  - open suspension procedures (to elevate the bladder neck to a position where intraabdominal pressure transmission is identical to that transmitted to the bladder)
  - sling procedures (to restore the suburethral 'hammock support'):
    - autologous
    - xenograft
    - cadaveric (allograft).
  - tape procedures (to restore the suburethral hammock support):
    - retropubic
    - transobturator
    - mini-slings.
  - artificial urinary sphincter (AUS), which can be useful in ISD.

Note that dual serotonin–noradrenaline reuptake inhibition therapies such as duloxetine are no longer recommended as first-line therapies owing to the severe side effects that can occur.

Urodynamics in stress incontinence

Voiding diaries – These are particularly useful in those with mixed symptoms suggestive of stress and urgency incontinence. They are useful if leakage (urgency vs. stress) is recorded to document the frequency of stress incontinence episodes. Prior to performing invasive urodynamics, a voiding diary will give an estimate of the bladder capacity, and this information should be used to prevent overfilling during the assessment. Many women with SUI alter their behaviour to try to cope better with the condition. For example, they may increase their urinary frequency to maintain an empty or low-volume bladder and thereby reduce the frequency or severity of any stress incontinence.

1-hour pad test – This test is useful in patients strongly suspected of urinary incontinence but who have failed to demonstrate any leakage on other investigations, such as video urodynamic studies. The test gives a quantification of the degree of incontinence.

Uroflowmetry – Uroflowmetry is not a particularly useful test in this condition, although it may be beneficial in ruling out any voiding dysfunction which may complicate treatment. Testing should be performed prior to pressure/flow cystometry to provide a representative indication of the voiding pattern that is likely to be encountered during invasive cystometry. An exaggerated flow rate or 'fast void' may be seen in patients with significant urethral insufficiency.

Pressure/flow cystometry – Video urodynamics is the gold standard test and allows leakage to be visualized with increases in intraabdominal pressure. In addition, bladder neck opening and bladder neck descent/hypermobility can also be assessed during screening. In the simplest of cases where there are no uncertainties regarding the diagnosis and no complicating factors, pressure/flow assessment is not required prior to surgery, although this recommendation remains controversial, and a diagnosis made based on history alone will not predict DO in up to 25% of cases. In all other cases, urodynamic testing should be performed to confirm the diagnosis, rule out other causes for the incontinence such as urgency incontinence or cough-provoked incontinence and assess for possible postoperative complications. For example, poor voiding function may suggest a potential need for CISC following an invasive procedure. Cystometry is recommended when considering an invasive procedure in patients who have had unsuccessful attempts at anti-incontinence surgery previously.

Other urodynamic tests – Electromyography measurement during pressure/flow studies may give an indication of the pelvic floor and/or sphincter activity. Urethral pressure profilometry measurement (Chapter 3) and abdominal leak point pressure (ALPP) (Chapter 4) may help determine if ISD is the cause of the SUI and possibly direct further management.

Possible findings during urodynamic testing of patients with stress incontinence	
Voiding diaries	• Episodes of stress incontinence, if recorded • Frequency as a coping behaviour
1-Hour pad test	• >1.4-g increase in weight
Uroflowmetry	• Possible exaggerated flow rate due to low outlet resistance
Pressure/flow cystometry	• Demonstrable urodynamic stress incontinence • Bladder neck descent and hypermobility • Suggests intrinsic sphincteric deficiency (video urodynamics) • Voiding usually rapid with a high flow rate (30–60 mL/s) and low voiding pressures due to reduced outflow resistance (see Fig. 5.10)
Electromyography	• Possibly demonstrates weakening of the pelvic floor
Urethral pressure profilometry	• Suggests intrinsic sphincteric deficiency
Abdominal leak point pressures	• Suggest intrinsic sphincteric deficiency

Table 5.2 *Possible findings during urodynamic testing of patients with stress incontinence.*

However, all of these tests are nonstandardized and currently provide data of uncertain clinical significance (Table 5.2).

Nonurodynamic tests – Cystoscopy adds little to the evaluation of patients who have stress incontinence, but it is occasionally helpful in assessing the short fibrotic 'stove-pipe' urethra sometimes present in patients who have ISD. Complex patients suspected of having a urogenital fistula or urethral diverticulum require an appropriate diagnostic workup, including cystoscopy.

Urodynamic findings in stress incontinence

Video urodynamics

Bladder neck descent and hypermobility – When the bladder descends due to poor pelvic floor support, increases in intraabdominal pressure are not transmitted equally to the bladder body and proximal urethra (Figs 5.10 and 5.11). Most of the increased pressure is transmitted only to the bladder. This elevates the intravesical pressure above the maximum pressure exerted by the urethral sphincter mechanism, resulting in urinary leakage. This is easily visualized with video urodynamics; when standing partially obliquely the bladder neck position may be abnormally low (below the level of the upper third of the pubic symphysis), signifying loss of pelvic floor

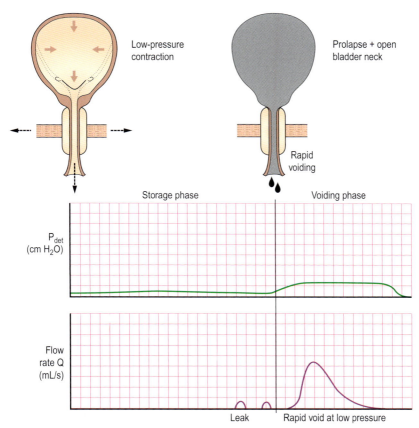

Fig. 5.10 *Typical video urodynamic appearances for urodynamic stress incontinence.* (**a**) *Video findings,* (**b**) *pressure flow findings. Low pressure, high flow due to decreased bladder outlet resistance and radiological evidence of an open bladder neck are shown.*

support. Coughing or a Valsalva causes the bladder and bladder neck to descend further, and leakage may become apparent (Fig. 5.12). On termination of the increased intraabdominal pressure, the bladder neck quickly 'springs back' to its original position, terminating leakage.

Whether to reduce a prolapse during a urodynamic study, both to compensate for the 'kinking'/'obstructive' effect of a cystourethrocoele and to replicate the effect of a surgical procedure, is often discussed and remains the subject of debate but limited consensus.

Intrinsic sphincter deficiency – With ISD the sphincter mechanism is weakened and therefore unable to resist the increases in intravesical

119

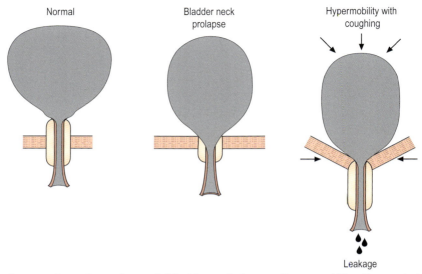

Normal

Bladder neck prolapse

Hypermobility with coughing

Leakage

Fig. 5.11 Stress incontinence in bladder neck descent/hypermobility. *There is a lack of transmission of pressure to the urethra, resulting in leakage.*

a

b

Fig. 5.12 Radiological appearances of bladder neck descent. *(a)* Cystogram of a *female patient in the supine position showing a degree of bladder base prolapse. (b) The same patient on coughing, showing descent of the bladder base and urethra; on the dynamic screening image, leakage was visible.*

Contributory causes to intrinsic sphincter deficiency	
Mechanism	**Causes**
Urethral trauma	Pelvic fracture, traumatic childbirth
Neurological disorder	Myelomeningocele, conus injuries of the cord
Vaginal delivery	Pudendal nerve injury
Previous operation	Failed operation for incontinence, urethral dilatation, urethral diverticulectomy, radical prostatectomy, radiotherapy

Table 5.3   *Intrinsic sphincter deficiency: contributory causes.*

pressure that occur with stress (Table 5.3). When ISD occurs in severe forms, even the slightest increase in pressure (e.g. from minor movement) may cause leakage or the sphincter may be completely open (incompetent) with almost continual leakage. Many patients are unable to interrupt micturition due to weakness of their striated sphincter mechanism. Unfortunately, there is no consensus regarding how best to assess for ISD, with advocates for physical examination (Q-tip test), video urodynamics, urethral pressure measurements and ALPP measurements (ALPP >100 cm H_2O is unlikely to be ISD; ALPP <60 cm H_2O is suggestive of ISD). This area needs further research, particularly with recent developments in therapies aimed specifically at treating ISD as opposed to bladder neck descent/hypermobility. However, in our opinion (based on current evidence), video urodynamics is essential to differentiate between the relative contributions of bladder neck prolapse/hypermobility and ISD, because it deals with function, anatomy and dynamics. Typically, on video urodynamics, patients with pure ISD demonstrate severe leakage with minimal increase in intraabdominal pressure, there is minimal bladder neck descent and the urethra does not spring back but appears to stay open and continues leaking even after the stress event. Often there is a rectangular-shaped incompetent bladder neck (Fig. 5.13), and this should be differentiated from the beaking of the bladder neck that is probably a normal finding, even in continent females.

OTHER TYPES OF INCONTINENCE

Mixed urinary incontinence – This is the complaint of involuntary leakage associated with urgency and also with exertion, effort, sneezing or coughing. Therefore it is a combination of:
- urgency incontinence and
- stress incontinence.

121

Fig. 5.13 *Screening appearances of intrinsic sphincter deficiency.* Cystourethrogram *showing a typical female patient with intrinsic sphincter deficiency and a well-supported bladder base with contrast on coughing filling the 'rectangular' urethra, with associated leakage.*

This problem is particularly common and presents a management dilemma, as patients are often refractory to initial treatments and certain treatments may aggravate the other component of the incontinence. For example, treating the stress component with an invasive procedure may aggravate the urgency incontinence component. Patients with mixed incontinence symptoms should ideally undergo video urodynamics to determine which component predominates and is associated with the most troublesome symptoms. Treating the most troublesome component first usually achieves the best long-term results, and often a variety of treatments is needed to optimize management.

Overflow incontinence – This is the involuntary loss of urine associated with overdistension of the bladder secondary to inefficient bladder emptying. It may occur as a result of:
- poor detrusor contractility
- BOO
- a combination of poor detrusor contractility and BOO.

Overflow incontinence is often seen in elderly men with chronic retention. Patients with inefficient bladder emptying and overdistension may present with unconscious dribbling, urinary frequency, urgency or SUI. For this reason, determination of the postvoid residual urine volume is important in all patients with urinary incontinence to exclude a diagnosis of chronic retention.

Nocturnal enuresis – This is the involuntary leakage of urine that occurs during sleep. The condition can be either primary (i.e. childhood), persistent primary (NE does not settle after childhood) or recurrent (NE returns after a period of absence). NE can occur alone, where it is termed *monosymptomatic nocturnal enuresis*, or in combination with other storage LUTS, where it is termed *nonmonosymptomatic nocturnal enuresis*. Primary forms of mono-symptomatic NE usually settle with behavioural therapies or simple pharmacotherapy alone, whilst nonmonosymptomatic NE is commonly associated with DO. It must be borne in mind that the recurrence of NE in the elderly can indicate chronic retention associated with high bladder pressures and upper tract decompensation.

Unconscious incontinence – This is unperceived involuntary incontinence of urine, neither related to abdominal straining nor associated with urgency. The patient's first sensation is wetness. Its identification is important because it usually represents marked bladder dysfunction.

Most patients who have unconscious incontinence have either:
- significant ISD
- DO not perceived as urgency because of poor bladder sensation (commonly seen in elderly patients and in those who have neuropathic bladders)
- overflow incontinence (see earlier discussion).

Situational urinary incontinence – This category includes types of urinary incontinence that only occur in certain situations, and they may be related to underlying stress incontinence or underlying DO, such as that occurring during sexual intercourse or during giggling, often called *giggle incontinence* (Fig. 5.14).

Continuous urinary incontinence – This is the complaint of continuous leakage of urine. It may be due to a urogenital fistula (e.g. a vesicovaginal fistula), a congenital abnormality (e.g. an ectopic ureter) or possibly due to gross ISD. Some elderly patients with significant urethral insufficiency and/or severe DO report leaking 'all the time'.

123

Fig. 5.14 *Giggle incontinence. Detrusor overactivity provoked by giggling is shown.*

Coexistence of different types of incontinence – Any of the types of incontinence described previously can exist in combination. As with mixed incontinence, identification of the various contributory factors are important because they influence treatment selection and help in anticipating postoperative problems. Video urodynamics in combination with a thorough urological history and physical examination forms the cornerstone of the evaluation of these more complex patients.

INCONTINENCE IN MEN

Urinary incontinence is far less common in men due to the much more adequate urethral/sphincter mechanism. Most cases of male incontinence are due to:

- DO
- neurogenic lower urinary tract dysfunction
- post-prostatectomy (particularly radical prostatectomy)
- overflow incontinence.

Urodynamics forms the cornerstone for evaluating male voiding dysfunction. Indications for pressure/flow cystometry include:

- any type of urinary incontinence
- suspected urethral sphincter insufficiency
- poor voiding function combined with marked storage symptoms
- chronic retention
- recurrent symptoms following surgery
- patients with known or suspected neurological dysfunction of the lower urinary tract
- younger patients (<55 years of age)
- storage LUTS refractory to medical therapy.

POST-PROSTATECTOMY INCONTINENCE

Urinary incontinence can be one of the most debilitating and devastating complications following prostatectomy. Its incidence following transurethral resection of the prostate is less than 1%; however, following radical prostatectomy for prostate cancer the incidence of severe or total incontinence is approximately 2% to 12%, with up to 50% of patients complaining of milder stress leakage.

Usually during a prostatectomy the proximal urethral sphincter is ablated, and therefore continence is maintained only by the distal urethral sphincter, which is composed of both striated and smooth muscle components (see Chapter 2). However, if there is preexisting incompetence of the distal urethral sphincter or if it (or its innervation) is damaged by surgery, then incontinence may occur.

Predisposing causes of distal sphincteric damage before prostatectomy include:
- pelvic trauma
- denervation after radical pelvic surgery
- intervertebral disc disease
- radical radiotherapy.

Sphincteric incompetence resulting from surgery is usually due to:
- neural injury or sphincteric denervation
- periurethral fibrosis.

Because the intrinsic smooth muscle of the distal sphincter mechanism is separate from the extrinsic striated muscle of the periurethral pelvic floor, most patients with post-prostatectomy incontinence are able to stop and start their urinary stream using the periurethral striated muscles.

125

However, not all post-prostatectomy incontinence is secondary to distal sphincteric incompetence. Other causes include:

- DO with and without poor bladder compliance:
  - primary – present before the surgery but only becomes problematic as a consequence of the marked reduction in the integrity of the sphincter mechanisms
  - secondary – as a consequence of the surgery.
- BOO with overflow incontinence:
  - bladder neck contracture
  - urethral stricture.

DO may be present in up to 50% of patients who are incontinent following prostatectomy and may be the underlying cause of the incontinence or a significant contributing factor.

Patient evaluation in post-prostatectomy incontinence

Patients with incontinence following prostatectomy require an in-depth history and physical examination. Most patients give a history of stress incontinence and slow dribbling leakage when standing upright. Many patients are continent when supine and only experience stress or urgency incontinence when changing posture to the standing position. On examination, patients who have sphincteric incompetence often leak when asked to perform a Valsalva manoeuvre. Any abnormal neurology may suggest an underlying abnormality leading to sphincteric denervation. Overflow incontinence can also be excluded by suprapubic palpation and measuring a post-void residual. Urinalysis is necessary to exclude a urinary tract infection.

URODYNAMICS IN PRACTICE: POST-PROSTATECTOMY INCONTINENCE

- Pressure/flow cystometry is necessary for evaluating incontinence following prostatectomy.
- Cystometry will help establish a diagnosis of sphincteric incompetence if stress incontinence is present – a low abdominal leak point pressure of less than 60 cm H_2O correlates with sphincteric incompetence but is not diagnostic. Video urodynamics is particularly helpful.
- Cystometry will identify and characterize any detrusor dysfunction, which may be the cause of or a major contributory factor to the incontinence.
- Commonly, patients following prostatectomy demonstrate detrusor overactivity, bladder hypersensitivity or poor bladder compliance.
- Video urodynamics is particularly useful if there is any obstruction to identify the level of the obstruction.

- Measurement of the urethral pressure profile is of limited value and is generally not recommended.
- The urethral catheter may mask leakage in men with mild stress incontinence; in these cases the catheter should be removed and the abdominal pressure used to assess the Valsalva leak point.

Management

The therapeutic armamentarium for post-prostatectomy incontinence includes:
- behavioural therapy
- pelvic floor exercises
- anticholinergic or beta-3 pharmacotherapy (DO that cannot be controlled medically may be a poor prognostic indicator before insertion of an AUS)
- periurethral injection therapy
- AUS implantation
- male sling procedures.

The success rate for periurethral injection therapy is less than 30%. The treatment of choice for post-prostatectomy stress incontinence secondary to sphincteric incompetence is the AUS; approximately 90% of patients achieve social continence, and nearly 50% achieve complete continence. In experienced hands the AUS gives patients the highest chance of cure and should be offered to appropriate patients, whilst there has been increasing interest in the use of male sling procedures. The MASTER randomized controlled trial compares the AUS to the male sling for patients with post-prostatectomy incontinence, and the results of this trial are currently awaited.

CHAPTER 6

Voiding disorders and bladder outflow obstruction

INTRODUCTION

Due to the high prevalence of bladder outflow obstruction (BOO) secondary to benign (and malignant) prostatic disease, voiding difficulties are the most common reason men seek a urologist. However, recent evidence shows that a large proportion of men have a storage disorder such as overactive bladder either as a primary diagnosis or secondary to BOO. Considering that voiding disorders frequently are associated with storage lower urinary tract symptoms (LUTS) such as nocturia and daytime frequency, this may well lead to a confusing mix of symptoms. With this in mind, men with LUTS should not be assumed to have a voiding disorder/prostatic disease, and if there is any doubt as to the diagnosis, then pressure/flow cystometry is necessary to differentiate definitively between voiding and storage disorders.

Causes of voiding difficulty in men are:

- **Anatomical outflow obstruction:**
  ○ obstruction at the level of the prostate (most common)
  ○ obstruction at the level of the bladder neck
  ○ obstruction due to a urethral stricture
  ○ extrinsic compression of bladder or urethra (e.g. from a tumour).
- **Functional obstruction:**
  ○ overactivity of the bladder neck/urethral muscles causing dyssynergy with the detrusor contraction.
- **Detrusor underactivity:**
  ○ primary
  ○ secondary to outflow obstruction or a neurogenic disorder.

Voiding difficulty is far less common in females, and when it occurs it should be thoroughly investigated with anatomical and functional investigations. Most female patients with voiding difficulty have a neuropathic disorder affecting the bladder, but a functional obstruction of the bladder

129

outlet/urethra or detrusor muscle failure must be excluded. Causes of voiding difficulty in women are:

- **Anatomical outflow obstruction:**
  - overcorrection following cystourethropexy
  - extrinsic compression of bladder/neck urethra (e.g. from a tumour or pelvic organ prolapse)
  - obstruction at the level of the bladder neck
  - urethral stenosis (stricture).
- Functional obstruction:
  - overactivity of the bladder neck/urethral muscles causing dyssynergy with the detrusor contraction.
- **Detrusor underactivity:**
  - primary
  - secondary to outflow obstruction or a neurogenic disorder.
- **Small-volume urinary frequency:**
  - many women with bladder overactivity report symptoms such as poor flow and hesitancy as a result of voiding prematurely at low bladder urine volumes.

ANATOMICAL BLADDER OUTFLOW OBSTRUCTION

Bladder outflow obstruction is a generic term for obstruction during voiding and is characterized by increased detrusor pressure and reduced urine flow rate. It is usually diagnosed definitively during pressure/flow cystometry, although history, physical evaluation and simple urodynamic tests such as voiding diaries, uroflowmetry and postvoid residual (PVR) often point to the correct diagnosis; most patients do not undergo pressure/flow cystometry until initial treatment has failed or until there are other complicating factors.

Most patients present with predominant voiding LUTS, but some present with complications of BOO, including:

- acute urinary retention
- chronic urinary retention
- renal impairment and hydronephrosis
- urinary tract infections
- bladder calculi
- haematuria
- secondary detrusor overactivity. (Note: This occurs in up to 70% of men with prostatic BOO; it resolves in up to two-thirds of patients following surgical relief of the obstruction, although this suggests a causal relationship between BOO and detrusor overactivity in many patients; recent work has challenged this apparent causal link.)

Benign prostatic obstruction

TERMINOLOGY: ENLARGEMENT OF THE PROSTATE

Benign prostatic hyperplasia (BPH): A histological diagnosis present in up to 50% of men older than 60 years and nearly 88% by 80 years. The extent to which prostatic enlargement and symptoms secondary to BPH manifest themselves is variable.

Benign prostatic enlargement (BPE): Prostatic enlargement due to histological BPH. This term should be used when clinically detectable prostatic enlargement is evident in the absence of a known histological diagnosis of BPH.

Benign prostatic obstruction (BPO): Obstruction to urinary flow demonstrable on pressure/flow cystometry secondary to the prostate gland. This may be due to enlargement of the prostate gland (Fig. 6.1a) or to increased prostatic smooth muscle tone causing contraction of the prostate gland around the prostatic urethra (therefore the prostate does not need to be particularly enlarged to cause obstruction!).

Treatment options include:
- **Conservative measures:**
  - fluid intake advice
  - improve mobility/dexterity/mental state.
- **Phytotherapy** (alternative medications from plant extracts; not recommended by World Health Organization consensus).
- **α1-Adrenoceptor antagonists:**
  - alfuzosin
  - doxazosin
  - tamsulosin
  - terazosin
  - silodosin.
- **5-Alpha reductase inhibitors:**
  - finasteride
  - dutasteride
- **Combination therapy of α1-adrenoceptor antagonists and 5-alpha reductase inhibitors**
- **Emerging potential medication choices for male LUTS:**
  - anticholinergics, alone or in combination with α1-adrenoceptor antagonists
  - beta-3 adrenoreceptor agonists, alone or in combination with α1-adrenoceptor antagonists
  - Phosphodiesterase type 5 inhibitors, alone or in combination with α1-adrenoceptor antagonists.

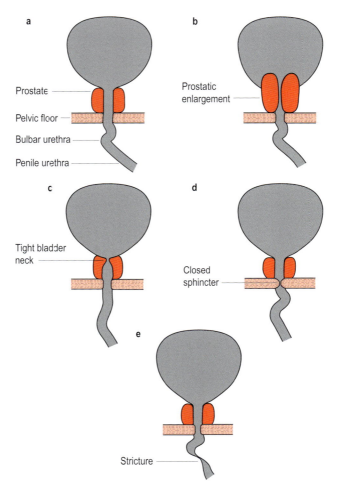

Fig. 6.1 *Screening appearances of bladder outflow obstruction.* *(**a**) Normal appearance of male lower urinary tract during voiding. (**b**) Prostatic obstruction: lengthening and thinning of prostatic urethra, prostatic indentation of the bladder neck. (**c**) Bladder neck obstruction: bladder neck shut or narrow during voluntary voiding contraction. (**d**) Detrusor sphincter dyssynergia: narrow membranous urethra, bulging of prostatic urethra. (**e**) Urethral stricture.*

- **Invasive treatments:**
  - *Prostatectomy (usually transurethral resection of the prostate [TURP]).* The use of TURP has declined in recent years due to the efficacy of medications in reducing symptoms and preventing progression. A variety of methods of performing prostatectomy or ablation of the prostate gland have been described, including high-intensity ultrasound,

microwave thermotherapy, needle ablation, electrovaporization and laser therapy. Open retropubic prostatectomy is also used in particularly large prostates, in which the open operation is quicker and safer than TURP. Prostatectomy is more successful in patients with demonstrable BOO on pressure/flow cystometry than in patients without documented obstruction.

○ *Transurethral incision of the prostate (bladder neck).* Generally used for smaller prostates, the procedure has less associated morbidity than prostatectomy.

○ *Open retropubic prostatectomy.* Occasionally appropriate for large prostates, this is an effective surgical approach that is now rarely used.

○ *Laser or electrosurgical enucleation of the prostate.* This procedure is recognized to have a steep learning curve but is considered to potentially provide a more pronounced relief of obstruction; it is similar to open prostatectomy.

○ *Laser ablation of the prostate (green light).* This procedure offers good haemostasis and in experienced hands provides similar initial results to transurethral resection or incision of the prostate.

○ *Prostatic stents.* These stents have been used in elderly men not fit for surgery, who do not wish to be catheterized for a long term; however, stents have a very limited role and are associated with significant morbidity.

○ *Minimally invasive approaches (including insertion of prostatic UroLift implants and water ablation of the prostate).* These therapies are currently at a trial stage and are not recommended for those with an obstructing middle lobe.

Catheterization to drain the bladder either with an indwelling catheter or clean intermittent self-catheterization (CISC) may be required in patients who are refractory to conservative or medical treatments and in those who are not fit or are unwilling to undergo an invasive procedure.

CLINICAL NOTE: BENIGN PROSTATIC DISEASE

- Evaluation of a male patient includes obtaining an appropriate history and physical examination, in addition to urinalysis, laboratory tests and uroflowmetry.
- Treatment is directed at improving quality of life, relieving bladder outflow obstruction and resolving its complications.
- Watchful waiting and pharmacotherapy tend to be the choice of therapies for mild to moderate symptoms.
- Transurethral resection of the prostate remains the gold standard technique, but there has been a dramatic decline in the number of procedures performed due to the increasing use of effective medication.

Malignant prostatic obstruction

Benign and malignant prostatic diseases often coexist, but the relationship appears to be coincidental; however, both conditions are under the influence of the male hormone testosterone:

- Carcinoma usually originates in the peripheral zone.
- Benign prostatic enlargement usually originates in the central periure-thral zone.

Prostatic carcinoma must be excluded in middle-aged and elderly men who present with storage or voiding LUTS. If carcinoma is discovered, it must be treated appropriately depending on the grade and stage of the disease and the medical condition of the patient, as per relevant guidelines. Initial screening during assessment of LUTS is usually with digital rectal examination (DRE) and serum prostate-specific antigen (PSA), followed by transrectal ultrasound and prostatic biopsy if there is any suspicion of carcinoma.

Bladder neck obstruction

In this condition the bladder neck does not open completely during voiding, and there is little or no flow during a well-sustained detrusor contraction. Video urodynamics is necessary to make the diagnosis (see Fig. 6.1c). The condition is especially prevalent in younger men and also occurs occasionally in women; currently the aetiology of pri-mary bladder neck obstruction is unknown. Theories for the cause include fibrosis, neurogenic dysfunction (detrusor/bladder neck dyssy-nergia) and smooth muscle hypertrophy, amongst others. On screening, there may be trapping of contrast during the stop test (Fig. 6.2; see Fig. 4.20).

Treatment of bladder neck obstruction includes:

- watchful waiting
- α1-adrenoceptor antagonists:
  - ○ alfuzosin
  - ○ doxazosin
  - ○ tamsulosin
  - ○ terazosin
  - ○ silodosin.
- transurethral incision of the bladder neck.

Fig. 6.2 *Bladder neck obstruction/dyssynergia.* *Trapping of contrast in the prostatic urethra during a stop test is shown. During voiding the patient is instructed to stop his urinary stream. Normally the contrast located in the prostatic urethra quickly milks back into the bladder; however, in patients with bladder neck dyssynergia, the tighter bladder neck resists retrograde flow, resulting in 'ballooning' of the prostatic urethra.*

CLINICAL NOTE: POST MICTURITION DRIBBLE

The symptom of post-micturition dribble is usually not due to obstruction but results from pooling of urine in the bulbar urethra and is common:

- if there is bladder neck obstruction
- in association with a urethral stricture or following urethroplasty
- with increasing age, presumably due to loss of elasticity of the urethra.

Urethral stricture

Urethral strictures can occur in men of all ages, and symptoms tend to only become evident when the urethral calibre is reduced to below 11 French. Strictures prevent the urethra from expanding and cause a characteristic constrictive picture on uroflowmetry (see Fig. 3.4e).

Causes of urethral stricture include:

- urethral trauma (e.g. injury, catheterization, surgery)
- urethral infection (usually sexually transmitted diseases)
- urethral inflammation
- urethral tumour (rare).

Although pressure/flow cystometry is useful in confirming BOO, more useful investigations include urethrography and cystoscopy, which provide an anatomical assessment of the stricture (see Fig. 6.1e). Treatment is essentially surgical, usually with urethrotomy for simple short strictures or a urethroplasty for long, complex or recurrent strictures. Patients may require

135

temporary bladder drainage via a catheter whilst awaiting surgery or if the surgery fails. Urethral dilatation is also helpful to maintain urethral patency both prior to and following surgery.

Evaluation of suspected bladder outflow obstruction

Initial evaluation of anatomical BOO includes:

- **History:**
  - character of symptoms (voiding versus storage)
  - severity of symptoms:
    - usually using a symptom score such as the International Prostate Symptom Score (IPSS) or American Urological Association Symptom Index (AUA-SI) (Fig. 6.3)
    - impact on quality of life.
  - previous treatments
  - current medications
  - comorbidities.
- **Examination:**
  - abdomen for masses and palpable bladder
  - DRE for prostatic enlargement and signs of malignancy.
- **Investigations:**
  - urine dipsticks and/or midstream urine culture to rule out haematuria, pyuria or infection
  - PSA to screen for carcinoma and as a proxy for prostate size (only following appropriate counselling of the patient)
  - uroflowmetry for characteristic pattern of poor voiding
  - PVR to assess for raised residuals or retention
  - serum urea and electrolytes to assess renal function
  - voiding diary to assess frequency and nocturia.

Further investigations should be performed if indicated, including (but not limited to):
- pressure/flow cystometry
- abdominal/renal ultrasonography
- transrectal ultrasonography and prostatic biopsy
- cystoscopy
- urethrography.

Indications for urodynamics to assess bladder outflow obstruction

Voiding diaries – These are helpful in quantifying the symptoms of urgency, frequency and nocturia which are commonly associated with BOO and also

International Prostate Symptom Score (IPSS) *(Please circle the appropriate score)*

	Not at all	Less than 1 time in 5	Less than half the time	About half the time	More than half the time	Almost always
1. Since the last visit, how often have you had a sensation of not emptying your bladder completely after you finished urinating?	0	1	2	3	4	5
2. Since the last visit, how often have you had to urinate again less than two hours after you finished urinating?	0	1	2	3	4	5
3. Since the last visit, how often have you found you stopped and started again several times when you urinated?	0	1	2	3	4	5
4. Since the last visit, how often have you found it difficult to postpone urination?	0	1	2	3	4	5
5. Since the last visit, how often have you had a weak urinary stream?	0	1	2	3	4	5
6. Since the last visit, how often have you had to push or strain to begin urination?	0	1	2	3	4	5
	None	1 time	2 times	3 times	4 times	5 or more times
7. Since the last visit, how many times did you most typically get up to urinate from the time you went to bed at night until the time you got up in the morning?	0	1	2	3	4	5

Total IPSS Score =

Quality of life due to urinary symptoms *(Please circle the appropriate score)*

	Delighted	Pleased	Mostly satisfied	Mixed (about equally satisfied and dissatisfied)	Mostly dissatisfied	Unhappy	Terrible
1. If you were to spend the rest of your life with your urinary condition just the way it is now, how would you feel about that?	0	1	2	3	4	5	6

Quality of life assessment score =

Fig. 6.3 International Prostate Symptom Score. *This questionnaire is commonly used in the assessment of benign prostatic disease.*

occur in storage disorders such as overactive bladder. They may also be useful in ruling out suspected nocturnal polyuria, particularly when the patient complains of significant nocturia (see Chapter 3).

Uroflowmetry and postvoid residual – These tests can be used as a screening tool, and in most cases are all that is required to confirm the presence of BOO (although it cannot exclude the presence of detrusor underactivity [DU]) before initiating treatment. In addition, it is a simple noninvasive test that can be used for subsequent monitoring following therapy. Urethral strictures produce a characteristic pattern (see Fig. 3.4e) due to the constrictive obstruction, which may aid in making the diagnosis of stricture disease.

Pressure/flow cystometry – During voiding, abnormally high pressures accompanied by a poor and prolonged urinary flow are characteristic of BOO. Cystometry is particularly useful in equivocal patients when it is necessary to rule out a detrusor cause for the LUTS, such as detrusor overactivity during the storage phase, or another cause for the dysfunctional voiding, such as DU during the voiding phase. It is also important that any patient being considered for further surgery after initial failed surgery undergoes pressure/flow cystometry, both to confirm that the symptoms are indeed due to BOO and to determine if any other complicating pathology is present, such as detrusor overactivity.

Video urodynamics – This is the gold standard investigation. Not only is all information obtained as for pressure/flow cystometry, but the added radiological screening allows the level of the obstruction to be determined. Enlargement of the prostate may be seen as a reduced calibre of the prostatic urethra and also as a prostatic indentation at the bladder base. Trapping of urine in the prostatic urethra due to bladder neck obstruction may also be visible during the stop test (Fig 6.2). Chronic changes to the bladder, such as trabeculation and diverticula, and vesicoureteric reflux during the high pressures generated by the bladder during voiding may also be seen (Table 6.1).

URODYNAMICS IN PRACTICE: PROSTATIC OBSTRUCTION

- Whilst there is a reasonable correlation between storage symptoms and detrusor overactivity, voiding symptoms correlate poorly with bladder outflow obstruction.
- In most cases uroflowmetry and PVR estimation are sufficient to confirm a diagnosis of bladder outflow obstruction.
- Flow rate will not be able to differentiate between high detrusor pressure with low flow or low detrusor pressure with low flow – this distinction is important because many patients who have an unsatisfactory result following previous prostatic surgery have low-pressure, low-flow voiding dysfunction.

- Normal voiding may be maintained during the early stages of obstruction by a compensatory increase in voiding detrusor pressure.
- A detailed urodynamic investigation is essential if the flow rate is equivocal or if previous surgery has not led to any improvement or has left residual symptoms such as urgency or incontinence.

Urodynamic findings in bladder outflow obstruction

Possible findings during urodynamic testing of patients with BOO	
Voiding diaries	Increased daytime frequency Nocturia
Uroflowmetry and PVR	Initial hesitancy Prolonged flow time and voiding time Low Q_{max} (<15 mL/s) Low average flow rate Prolonged time to maximum flow Prolonged declining termination of flow Intermittent flow Raised PVR Characteristic low flow rate, long plateau in urethral stricture
Pressure/flow cystometry (Figs. 6.4 and 6.5)	High opening pressure, prolonged opening time High maximum detrusor pressure (often $>60–100$ cm H_2O) High pressure at maximum flow High closing pressure Low Q_{max} (<15 mL/s) Raised PVR Prolonged flow time Intermittent flow Abdominal straining to aid voiding Stop test – the isometric pressure contraction is often high (>50 cm H_2O), rarely able to perform due to the force of the detrusor contraction
Video urodynamics	Level of obstruction Calibre of urethra Stop test – trapping in prostatic urethra due to bladder neck obstruction Vesicoureteric reflux Hydronephrosis Trabeculation Diverticula

Table 6.1 *Possible findings during urodynamic testing of patients with bladder outflow obstruction.* PVR, *Postvoid residual.*

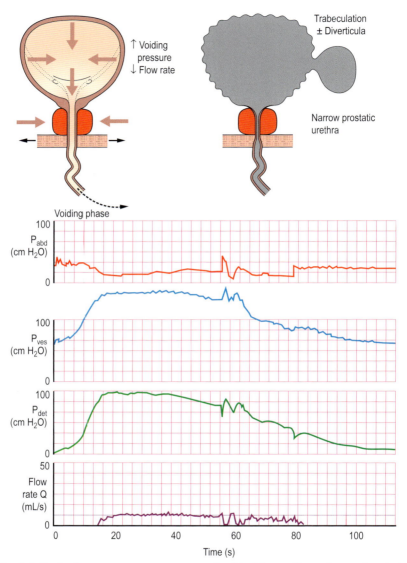

Fig. 6.4 *Typical cystometry appearances for bladder outflow obstruction.* In this case the screening schematic shows obstruction at the level of the prostate.

Fig. 6.5 *Pressure/flow trace in a patient with both detrusor overactivity during filling and bladder outflow obstruction during voiding.* This is a common pattern, as many patients have coexisting conditions.

Interpreting pressure/flow cystometry in bladder outflow obstruction

It is usually obvious during the voiding phase of a pressure/flow urodynamic investigation that BOO is present. Many experts regard patients with a detrusor pressure greater than 60 cm H_2O associated with a Q_{max} less than 10 mL/s to be urodynamically obstructed. The detrusor pressure often reaches abnormally high levels (approaching or >100 cm H_2O) in an attempt to expel the urine through the obstruction. Yet the flow rate remains low (often <8 mL/s) despite the elevated pressures (**high pressure, low flow**).

However, in many cases the findings are more equivocal, such as when:

- The elevated detrusor pressures with and without abdominal straining are able to overcome the obstruction leading to a normal flow rate (**high pressure, normal flow**).

141

- The detrusor has not yet accommodated to the BOO and generates only normal pressures; or the detrusor muscle is failing (but has not yet become hypocontractile, acontractile) and is only able to generate pressures in the normal range but no higher. The result with both of these scenarios is poor flow (**normal/low pressure, low flow**).

To aid in determining if BOO is present, the International Continence Society (ICS) pressure/flow nomogram can be used to calculate the bladder outflow obstruction index (BOOI) by plotting Q_{max} against $P_{det}@Q_{max}$. This will then categorize patients as being obstructed, unobstructed or equivocal. The ICS nomogram is based on several older nomograms (Abrams–Griffiths, Schafer LinPURR and URA) which were all found to have a high degree of correlation with each other, and therefore only the ICS nomogram is required in routine clinical practice (Fig. 6.6).

Modern urodynamic software usually contains the nomogram and will plot the data automatically; however, if the nomogram is unavailable the BOOI (previously called the *Abrams–Griffiths number*) can be easily calculated manually using the following formula:

$$BOOI = P_{det}@Q_{max} - (2 \times Q_{max})$$

$$BOOI < 20 = unobstructed$$

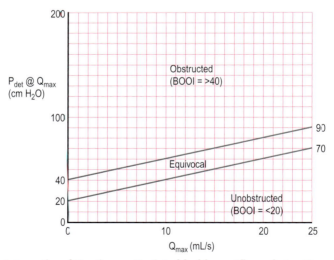

Fig. 6.6 *International Continence Society bladder outflow obstruction nomogram.* The nomogram allows the bladder outflow obstruction index to be easily calculated and the patient categorized as obstructed, unobstructed or equivocal. Adjustment must be made for flow rate delay before using the nomogram.

BOOI between 20 and 40 = equivocal

BOOI > 40 = obstructed

Example calculation:

If $P_{det}@Q_{max}$ is 100 cm H_2O and Q_{max} is 5 mL/s,

then the BOOI = $100 - (2 \times 5) = 90$ = obstructed.

When using the nomogram and/or calculating the BOOI, it must be remembered that the flow rate delay must be corrected when calculating the $P_{det}@Q_{max}$, and this will depend on the local characteristics of the equipment (see Chapter 4). It must also be borne in mind that the nomogram/ BOOI was developed to assess male BOO due to a presumed prostatic cause. The nomogram and BOOI may therefore not be applicable in other situations, such as in men with a functional obstruction (dyssynergia), and is not appropriate for women.

FUNCTIONAL OBSTRUCTION (DYSSYNERGIA)

During normal voiding the urethra relaxes synchronously with contraction of the detrusor muscle. If the urethra and particularly its associated sphincter mechanisms fail to relax during voiding, then uncoordinated activity between the detrusor and the urethra/sphincter occurs; this is termed *dyssynergia*. The ICS has defined several patterns of functional obstruction.

Dysfunctional voiding – 'An intermittent and/or fluctuating flow rate due to involuntary intermittent contractions of the peri-urethral striated muscle during voiding, in neurologically normal patients'. The condition occurs most frequently in children and is thought to be due to intermittent pelvic floor contractions. (The old term for this was *nonneurogenic, neurogenic bladder*.) Poor relaxation of the pelvic floor and urethral sphincter mechanism is also common in patients with voiding dysfunction, especially those with pelvic pain syndrome.

Detrusor sphincter dyssynergia (DSD) – 'A detrusor contraction concurrent with an involuntary contraction of the urethral and/or peri-urethral striated muscle' (see Fig. 6.1c). The condition tends to occur in patients with a suprasacral neurological lesion (e.g. a spinal cord injury), Parkinson's disease or multiple sclerosis (see Chapter 9). Coexisting DSD and prostatic obstruction can occur in elderly men, such as those with Parkinson's disease, and can be particularly difficult to manage. A useful therapeutic manoeuvre in such a situation can be to insert a temporary intraurethral prostatic stent to treat the prostate obstruction, thus allowing the two conditions to be differentiated.

Nonrelaxing urethral sphincter obstruction – 'A non-relaxing, obstructing urethra resulting in reduced urine flow' which tends to occur in patients with a sacral or infrasacral neurological lesion (e.g. meningo-myelocoele) or following radical pelvic surgery which has damaged the innervation.

Fowler's syndrome – This is an uncommon condition that primarily affects young women in their 20s to 30s, in whom the urethral sphincter mechanism fails to relax, leading to raised PVRs and retention. There may be a history of lifelong voiding difficulty, and often there is associated secondary detrusor failure. Many of these women have an associated hormonal problem (Stein–Leventhal syndrome – hirsutism, polycystic ovary syndrome and amenor-rhoea). The aetiology is unknown, and the gold standard investigation for this condition is sphincter electromyography (EMG), although pressure/flow cystometry, urethral pressure profilometry and ultrasound sphincter volume measurement may also be valuable. Some women may spontane-ously recover, whilst in others it may be a lifelong condition. CISC may be required to ensure adequate bladder drainage, although it is poorly correlated, and sacral neuromodulation has also been found to be of some benefit in restoring a voiding pattern.

Evaluation of suspected functional obstruction

The preceding brief descriptions should be borne in mind when evaluating any patient who has outflow obstruction. Associated neurological symp-toms and signs should suggest the possibility of DSD or a nonrelaxing urethral sphincter obstruction.

These conditions are best evaluated using video urodynamics with synchronous use of EMG and should ideally be performed in units with specialist expertise in investigating and managing these conditions.

Urodynamic findings in functional obstruction

Urodynamic findings are similar to those seen in anatomical BOO and are characterized by high detrusor pressures coupled with poor flow. With DSD the sphincter may intermittently open and close during void-ing. When the sphincter is open, the detrusor pressures may be normal or moderately high. If the sphincter suddenly closes during a void, the detrusor pressure rises because the detrusor is now isovolumetrically contracting against the closed sphincter (similar to a stop test); the flow rate will also reduce/stop whilst the sphincter is closed. When the sphincter reopens, the detrusor pressures will drop and the flow will be reestablished. This pattern may be repeated several times during a void (Fig. 6.7).

Video urodynamics will also show the intermittent sphincter activity and the level of the obstruction. In addition, the bladder may develop chronic

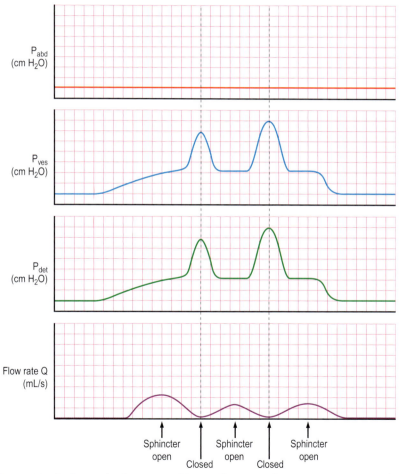

Fig. 6.7 Typical trace in detrusor sphincter dyssynergia. *Intermittent opening and closure of the urethral sphincter, causing a characteristic flow pattern and pressure changes.*

145

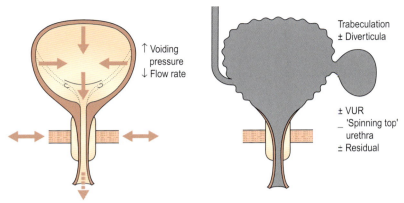

Fig. 6.8 Video appearances of detrusor sphincter dyssynergia. *High pressure and low flow from sphincter obstruction may lead to chronic changes. VUR, Vesicoureteric reflux.*

changes due to the elevated voiding pressures, including trabeculation, diverticula and vesicoureteric reflux (most noticeable when the sphincter closes, causing a significant rise in detrusor pressure). The bladder and urethra in females may develop a 'spinning top' appearance due to widening of the posterior urethra from the chronic high-pressure trapping of urine in the urethra above the sphincter when the sphincter closes (Fig. 6.8). EMG studies concurrent with pressure/flow cystometry may also show intermittent sphincteric activity during voiding.

DETRUSOR UNDERACTIVITY AND THE UNDERACTIVE BLADDER

In addition to anatomical or functional obstruction to the bladder outflow, poor detrusor function can also lead to voiding dysfunction in both men and women. The urodynamic finding of an impaired detrusor contraction during the voiding phase is termed *detrusor underactivity*. The symptoms that occur as a consequence of DU could be categorized as those of the underactive bladder (see Chapter 4).

Poor detrusor function during voiding can be classified as:

- **Detrusor underactivity** – where the contraction of the detrusor is of reduced strength and/or duration, resulting in prolonged bladder emptying and/or failure to achieve complete bladder emptying within a normal time span. This was previously termed *hypocontractile detrusor*.
- **Acontractile detrusor** – where the detrusor cannot be demonstrated to contract during urodynamic assessment. This is a distinct entity from the inability to void during pressure/flow studies, which is a common occurrence.

Causes of detrusor underactivity failure include:
- **Primary:**
  - ○ idiopathic.
- **Secondary:**
  - ○ neurogenic bladder dysfunction (usually lower motor neuron)
  - ○ BOO.

Patients with DU often demonstrate two distinct symptom patterns: those who demonstrate poor bladder emptying and complain of symptoms (both voiding and storage), and those with chronic retention. DU should be considered in all patients who present with voiding difficulty. However, often the first presenting symptoms of a patient with chronic retention may be those of nocturnal incontinence. An intermittent straining pattern or sometimes a prolonged, low flow rate void associated with a raised PVR should raise suspicions of DU (although a similar picture is frequently seen with BOO). Only pressure/flow cystometry can definitively differentiate between BOO and DU, and therefore such testing should be performed in all equivocal cases, especially if the PVR is abnormally raised.

Chronic retention – This is a nonpainful distended bladder, which remains palpable or percussible after the patient has passed urine.

Elderly men in particular are at risk of developing chronic retention secondary to BOO, but any of the causes of DU may lead to chronic retention. Usually the cause of the chronic retention is unknown (idiopathic). A small group of middle-aged to elderly women present with retention of urine, usually after surgery, and commonly vigorously deny any previous history of voiding difficulty. In addition, some women report 'chronic holding' either due to busy schedules or in an attempt to avoid public restrooms. Urodynamic investigation sometimes demonstrates an underactive detrusor with chronic retention in this distinct group.

Management of detrusor underactivity

Initial – The initial management of DU is aimed at ensuring that the bladder is adequately drained, thus preventing overdistension of the bladder and overstretching of the detrusor muscle fibres leading to further damage, and also preventing the development or worsening of damage to the upper urinary tracts. Abdominal voiding (i.e. Crede's manoeuvre) is not recommended due the excessively high vesical pressures that can be generated.

Bladder drainage can be achieved by:
- CISC – preferred option

- Indwelling catheterization:
  - urethral
  - suprapubic (preferable to long-term urethral catheterization), which is particularly useful in patients with a suspected reversible neurological disorder, as it allows the serial assessment of PVRs to assess the ability to void spontaneously.

Long term – The long-term management of DU is directed at the correction of any underlying aetiology, if possible. If the underlying cause is adequately treated and the bladder is allowed a period of 'rest' with suitable drainage, then there may be some recovery of detrusor function.

In a man with DU secondary to long-standing prostatic BOO, a period of drainage may allow detrusor function to improve. In such a situation, proceeding to prostatic surgery may be appropriate, whilst if there is no improvement in detrusor function, then the voiding symptoms are unlikely to resolve following outflow tract surgery and the man is likely to continue to need artificial bladder draining following prostatic surgery.

Urodynamics in detrusor underactivity

Uroflowmetry and postvoid residual – Uroflowmetry and PVR estimation are good screening tools for DU. In particular, the PVR should always be related to the voided volumes measured on a frequency volume chart. The ratio of the PVR/mean voided volume+PVR (functional capacity) is the so-called voiding efficiency, and expert opinion suggests that a voiding efficiency of 40% or less is acceptable (e.g. a residual of 100 mL with a functional capacity of 200 mL is 50% compared to a PVR of 100 mL and a functional capacity of 50 mL where the voiding efficiency is 20%).

A prolonged flow is usually seen along with a low Q_{max}. Often the flow is intermittent, and the patient may be attempting to void with abdominal straining. The PVR is commonly raised (usually >200–300 mL). The flow rate pattern may be similar to the pattern seen in BOO where there may also be a raised PVR, and it is impossible to be sure if voiding dysfunction is due to DU or BOO based on this test.

Pressure/flow cystometry – This testing will determine if DU is present. During the storage phase the bladder may be hyposensitive with raised volumes at first sensation of filling and bladder sensations at strong desire to void and with a raised cystometric capacity. However, the patient may not demonstrate a strong desire to void and thus may not have a measurable maximum cystometric capacity. On being given permission to void, the patient often has a long delay before initiating the void. The detrusor pressure only rises minimally (or not at all if acontractile) with a corresponding low flow rate (**low-pressure, low-flow voiding**). Often the patient has to perform abdominal straining to initiate or maintain a void. Frequently only a negligible amount of fluid is voided (Fig. 6.9). It is not

Fig. 6.9 *Typical video urodynamic appearances for an underactive detrusor. The trace shows virtually no detrusor activity. The patient has voided small amounts by intermittent abdominal straining.*

possible to comment on whether there is a relative degree of BOO if an adequate detrusor pressure is not generated. There is no consensus on the diagnostic criteria; however, many would consider a BOOI less than 20 and a bladder contractility index (BCI) less than 100 diagnostic, where the $BCI = P_{det}@Q_{max} + (5Q_{max})$. These indexes, however, do not consider the coexistence of BOO and DU, and therefore several mathematical calculations have been described, including the Watts factor, but these are not usually calculated in routine practice, and future work should be directed at evaluating this further.

Video urodynamics – This is useful to determine if there is any reflux of contrast to the upper tract at any point during the study and may also show hydronephrosis if there is any upper tract dilatation. Video urodynamics is particularly important in patients with suspected neurogenic dysfunction. If sufficient contrast is voided, then it may be possible to assess the outflow tract, and in the presence of low voiding detrusor pressures, it is difficult to evaluate the significance of attenuation of the prostatic urethra.

URODYNAMICS IN PRACTICE: DETRUSOR UNDERACTIVITY AND OUTLET RESISTANCE

It must be remembered that a *normal* detrusor contraction will be recorded as:

- high pressure if the outlet is obstructed
- normal pressure if there is normal outlet resistance
- low pressure if there is low outlet resistance.

Voiding efficiency is a useful concept, and the potential degree of outlet resistance needs to be borne in mind. Therefore patients with previously unrecognized detrusor underactivity may have a very low outlet resistance, as may occur if the sphincteric mechanisms are impaired.

A patient with a very low outlet resistance is likely to experience stress incontinence during the filling phase.

CHAPTER 7

Sensory disorders

INTRODUCTION

Urodynamic investigations were originally developed to study the 'motor' function of the lower urinary tract. However, in recent years it has been recognized that the sensory component of voiding function is frequently involved in the pathophysiology of common lower urinary tract disorders such as overactive bladder syndrome. Bladder sensation can be assessed using stimulating electrodes introduced through the urethra, but such techniques are used for research purposes rather than routine assessment.

Urodynamic investigations are not ideal techniques for evaluating sensory disorders, which can be very subjective, but do allow some sensory information to be obtained and enable the observer to:

- measure the sensory thresholds objectively
- exclude motor disorders.

Abnormalities of bladder sensation can be broadly categorized into:

- increased bladder sensation (hypersensitive)
- reduced bladder sensation (hyposensitive).

Hypersensitivity

Increased bladder sensation – This is defined, during filling cystometry, as an early first sensation of bladder filling (or an early desire to void) and/or an early strong desire to void, which occurs at low bladder volume and which persists.

Causes of hypersensitivity include:

- **idiopathic**
- **bladder or urethral inflammation:**
  - ◯ bacterial cystitis
  - ◯ urethritis
  - ◯ urethral syndrome

- post-irradiation cystitis
- cyclophosphamide cystitis
- chemical cystitis, including ketamine bladder.
- **chronic prostatitis**
- **bladder pain syndrome/painful bladder syndrome/interstitial cystitis (BPS/PBS/IC)**
- **bladder calculus**
- **bladder carcinoma.**

Bacterial cystitis is the most common cause; it is therefore important to ensure that there is no concurrent infection immediately before performing pressure/flow urodynamics, as the test will often exacerbate the urinary infection and will produce a falsely increased bladder sensitivity.

Evaluation of bladder hypersensitivity

Patients with bladder hypersensitivity frequently complain of storage symptoms and also suprapubic pain in association with bladder filling.

A full history is particularly important in the assessment of hypersensitive disorders of the bladder. Clinical features can include:

- **daytime frequency** – a prominent symptom for which bladder pain rather than impending incontinence is the trigger
- **urgency** – but rarely associated with incontinence
- **bladder pain** – usually relieved by voiding
- **dysuria**
- **dyspareunia** – a common symptom
- **haematuria** – requires full investigation of both the lower and upper urinary tracts.

The symptoms are usually chronic, often with a history of previous probable urinary tract infections; however, urine cultures frequently have not been performed or the urine has been found to be sterile. Antibiotics have usually been unhelpful in providing long-term relief from the symptoms. Women often report improvement at the end of their menstrual cycle, and many will have had a hysterectomy, perhaps for lower abdominal/pelvic pain, but with no obvious gynaecological pathology.

Examination may be unremarkable, but attention should be paid to the urethral meatus, which may be inflamed or show mucosal prolapse (a urethral caruncle). There may also be bladder tenderness, both suprapubically and on vaginal examination. A gentle bimanual examination will identify other pelvic pathology. The iliococcygeus muscle or pelvic side wall is often tender, and trigger points may be identified.

All cases require urinalysis and culture to rule out an active urinary tract infection or haematuria. Often other investigations are indicated to exclude other causes for the symptoms, including:

- urine cytology
- voiding diaries
- pressure/flow cystometry
- cystoscopy with and without biopsy
- abdominal/pelvic ultrasound (to rule out gynaecological disorders).

Investigations of bladder oversensitivity are often complex with the requirement to exclude several pathologies. Fig. 7.1 shows a possible management pathway for the investigation and management of this complex problem.

Management is also often difficult, and options for bladder hypersensitivity and suspected BPS/PBS/IC include:

- Cystoscopy and overdistension (pressure of 80–100 cm H_2O for 5 min) and bladder biopsies of any abnormality as appropriate – this procedure is both investigative and in some cases therapeutic. There is usually a rise in pulse rate and blood pressure in patients with bladder hypersensitivity under a light general anaesthetic; in addition, bleeding and nonspecific glomerulations can often be seen in the bladder following the distension.
- Urethral recalibration up to 42 French – may improve symptoms if there is an associated urethral hypersensitivity.
- Intravesical installations may be helpful in some patients:
  - heparinoid agents (either alone or in combination with lidocaine and bicarbonate)
  - steroids
  - hyaluronic acid
  - chondroitin.
- Self-help groups (local and national).
- Diet and fluid intake manipulation.
- Medications:
  - nonsteroidal antiinflammatories
  - analgesics
  - anticholinergics
  - antidepressants
  - antihistamines
  - H_2 antagonists
  - pentosan polysulphate sodium
  - corticosteroids.

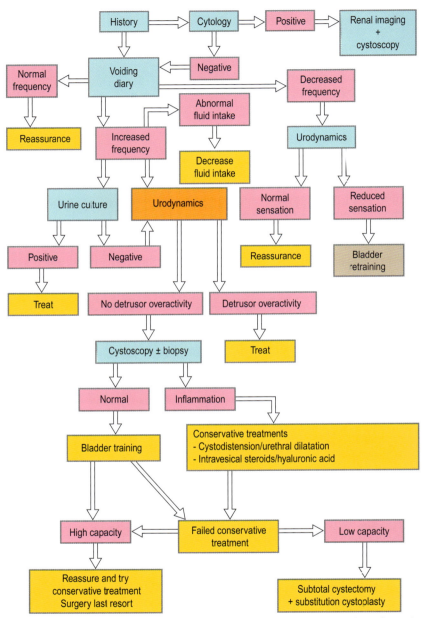

Fig. 7.1 *Algorithm for the management of hypersensitive bladder disorders.* *This is a complex area, and such an algorithm usually must be modified for each individual patient.*

- Surgery (if symptoms are intractable and debilitating):
  - cystectomy
  - enterocystoplasty.

It must be remembered that the evidence base for the clinical effectiveness of any of these therapies is very limited. Treatment of bladder hypersensitivity due to infection or mucosal inflammation is beyond the scope of this book.

Urodynamics in bladder hypersensitivity

The diagnosis of a hypersensitive bladder is one of exclusion, relying particularly on the exclusion of intravesical pathology, especially overt malignancy or carcinoma in situ.

Voiding diaries – Diaries are useful in this condition for determining the daytime frequency, which is often significantly raised; frequency typically is raised more than in patients with overactive bladder. However, the results often vary considerably from week to week, and it is essential to not base therapy on the results of voiding diaries alone.

Pressure/flow cystometry – This testing is particularly useful both in excluding other causes for the symptoms, including detrusor overactivity, and in diagnosing increased bladder sensation. Premature bladder sensations usually occur in quick succession, culminating in bladder discomfort and the strong desire to void, thereby reducing the capacity. In addition, patients with hypersensitive painful bladders often demonstrate high urethral closure pressures at rest and during voiding, increased electromyography activity with voiding and high voiding pressures.

URODYNAMICS IN PRACTICE: HYPERSENSITIVE BLADDER

- All patients who have symptoms suggestive of a hypersensitive bladder should have a urine culture; if negative, a urodynamic assessment is warranted.
- Urodynamics is helpful in diagnosing patients who have hypersensitive painful bladders and helps exclude other conditions, such as detrusor overactivity.
- Catheterization may be painful – passage of the catheter through the urethra and contact with the bladder mucosa may cause pain, suggesting the urethral syndrome.
- Major diagnostic features are premature first sensation of filling and premature first and strong desire to void. There is a reduced maximum cystometric capacity due to bladder discomfort.
- There is high voiding pressure associated with increased electromyography activity.

Continued

- Urethral pressure is high at rest and during voiding.
- Filling pressures and voiding function may be normal.
- The diagnosis of a 'hypersensitive bladder' is one of exclusion and relies on the exclusion of other intravesical pathologies, including malignancy.

HYPOSENSITIVE BLADDER

Reduced bladder sensation – This is defined, during filling cystometry, as diminished sensation throughout bladder filling.

Causes of hyposensitivity include:

- **idiopathic**
- **neurogenic:**
  - spinal cord injury
  - pelvic trauma
  - radical hysterectomy
  - abdominoperineal resection of the rectum
  - peripheral neuropathy (e.g. diabetes).
- **secondary:**
  - chronic retention and detrusor underactivity (see Chapter 6).

Due to the loss of desire to micturate, patients with a hyposensitive bladder often retain large volumes within the bladder and only infrequently void. This leads to chronic overdistension and eventually the development of detrusor underactivity. Conversely, detrusor underactivity due to other causes can also lead to painless chronic retention with resultant reduced bladder sensitivity. Therefore bladder hyposensitivity and underactive bladder frequently coexist and are intimately related (see Chapter 6).

Neurogenic hyposensitivity is usually due to denervation of the sensory pathways such as occurs with spinal cord injury or with local disruption to the nerves during pelvic surgery. Idiopathic hyposensitivity predominantly affects female patients with no other lower urinary tract pathology (and who commonly report 'holding' urination); this condition is sometimes referred to as 'camel bladder'.

Evaluation of bladder hyposensitivity

Patients who have a hyposensitive bladder often have no other symptoms apart from the loss of the desire to micturate. Other symptoms can include:

- straining to urinate with a poor flow

- a feeling of incomplete emptying
- infrequent voiding
- urinary frequency and incontinence secondary to poor bladder emptying
- recurrent urinary tract infections
- history of chronic retention.

There may also be a history of neurological injury (spinal cord or cauda equina), pelvic surgery or diabetes. Most patients with neurological trauma usually demonstrate a relative degree of detrusor underactivity.

Examination may reveal impaired sensation on testing the sacral dermatomes and raised postvoid residuals (PVRs).

Management of bladder hyposensitivity

It is important that the bladder is adequately drained to prevent the progression to an acontractile bladder or upper tract damage. Treatment choices are:

- **Bladder training** – If the patient can void spontaneously, then he or she should be encouraged to void 'by the clock' about six times a day and double void even though the desire to void may be absent. If such treatment is started early in the course of the condition, it may prevent subsequent impairment of detrusor function. It is important to monitor these patients carefully to check that they do not develop silent 'chronic retention' with increasing PVRs.
- **Alpha-adrenergic antagonists** – The success of alpha-adrenergic antagonists in improving the efficiency of voiding is limited, but empirical therapy may be of benefit.
- **Clean intermittent self-catheterization (CISC)** – If the patient is unable to initiate voiding or if voiding is inefficient with raised PVRs then CISC should be performed.

Urodynamics in bladder hyposensitivity

Voiding diaries – Diaries are useful in identifying infrequent voiding, and the patient's functional bladder capacity may be significantly increased. They may also be therapeutic when used in conjunction with bladder training.

Uroflowmetry and postvoid residual – This testing is not usually useful to investigate altered sensation; however, if there is any detrusor failure, then there may be poor voiding with a straining pattern and raised PVRs.

157

Pressure/flow cystometry – Diagnosis of hyposensitivity is dependent on increased volumes at which sensations occur; usually there is also a high cystometric capacity. There may be no strong desire to void, and often the urodynamicist will have to decide when to stop filling. In many cases there are no sensations felt throughout filling. If only hyposensitivity is present, then the voiding phase should be normal; however, if there is any associated detrusor underactivity, then voiding may be prolonged, intermittent and inefficient with no or minimal increase in detrusor pressure – a low-pressure, low-flow pattern (see Chapter 6).

URODYNAMICS IN PRACTICE: HYPOSENSITIVE BLADDER

- Characteristic urodynamic features are an increase in the volume at which the first sensation, first desire and strong desire to void occur, often with an associated high cystometric capacity.
- In severe cases there may be almost no bladder sensation, and thus voiding needs to be initiated without any desire to micturate 'by the clock'.
- In pure hyposensitivity, detrusor function during filling and voiding is normal.
- Detrusor underactivity may be a cause or consequence of bladder hyposensitivity and results in the inability to generate a detrusor contraction and often a high PVR.

CHAPTER 8

The contracted bladder

INTRODUCTION

Bladder contracture is the end stage of chronic inflammatory disorders of the bladder or results from the treatment of carcinoma such as that which occurs following radiotherapy. The chronic fibrotic damage to the bladder causes the bladder function to deteriorate severely.

Causes of fibrotic contracture include:

- prior bladder carcinoma treated by multiple resections
- surgery
- radiation therapy
- tuberculosis
- chemical cystitis, including the consequence of ketamine abuse
- severe sensory bladder disorders
- schistosomiasis.

Fibrotic contracture is often preceded by inflammation, so bladder hypersensitivity and contracture may coexist. However, the final stage of the condition may not be associated with hypersensitivity.

HISTORY AND EXAMINATION

The patient will usually have a previous long history of treatment for bladder carcinoma or chronic bladder inflammation. Symptoms of contracture can include:

- **daytime frequency and nocturia** – usually the predominant complaint
- **urgency** – often present
- **stress incontinence** – often present
- **bladder pain** – during filling if there is active inflammation of the bladder.

Examination is usually unremarkable, although there may be some suprapubic tenderness.

MANAGEMENT

In most cases, treatment of the underlying cause will have already failed to halt disease progression, and therefore operative treatment is indicated. Most cases of contracture are treated by cystectomy and urinary diversion or bladder reconstruction (see Chapter 5). More conservative treatments, such as cystodistension, do not produce long-term symptomatic relief.

Urodynamics in bladder contracture

Pressure/flow cystometry – Bladder contracture is best assessed with video urodynamics. Often during the filling phase, there is a reduction in the volumes at which bladder sensations, such as the first sensation of filling, occur and the maximum cystometric capacity is also reduced, giving the urodynamic appearance of bladder hypersensitivity. The compliance of the bladder is also often severely reduced due to fibrosis of the detrusor muscle (see Chapter 4). The findings must be interpreted in the context of data from a bladder diary and an assessment of anatomical bladder capacity.

In some instances there may be fibrosis around the bladder neck, thereby preventing adequate closure during filling and leading to incontinence. The incontinence may be due to the pressure rise in the bladder secondary to poor compliance or may be due to increased transmission of intraabdominal pressure (stress incontinence). In patients considering an enterocystoplasty, the outlet should be urodynamically assessed for the presence of intrinsic sphincter deficiency and the subsequent need for surgical correction at the time of bladder augmentation. Frequently there is fibrosis around the ureteric orifices, preventing closure, with resultant vesicoureteric reflux. In severe cases the upper tracts may act as a 'reservoir' for urine (with gross hydronephrosis) and may hold far more urine than the bladder.

Voiding may also be affected; fibrosis of the detrusor will lead to inefficient contractions and detrusor underactivity (see Chapter 6). The result will be a weak detrusor contraction coupled with a poor flow rate, prolonged voiding and raised postvoid residual (PVR); often the patient uses abdominal straining to aid voiding (low-pressure, low-flow voiding).

Video screening will not only determine if incontinence or vesicoureteric reflux is present but also usually shows that the bladder is small and unusually spherical in appearance (Fig. 8.1).

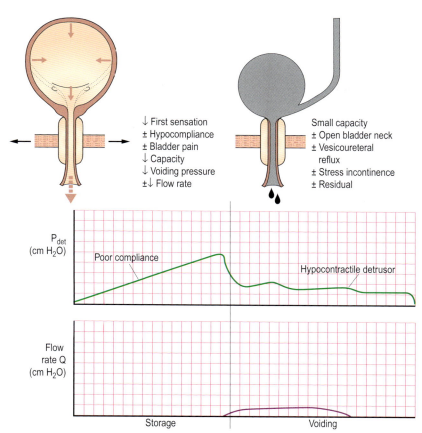

↓ First sensation
± Hypocompliance
± Bladder pain
↓ Capacity
↓ Voiding pressure
±↓ Flow rate

Small capacity
± Open bladder neck
± Vesicoureteral
   reflux
± Stress incontinence
± Residual

Fig. 8.1 *Typical urodynamic appearances for a contracted bladder.* The varied features that may be present on video urodynamics are summarized.

URODYNAMICS IN PRACTICE: THE CONTRACTED BLADDER

Frequent urodynamic findings include:
- reduction in first sensation volume
- reduction in first desire and strong desire volume
- reduced cystometric capacity
- reduced bladder compliance
- incontinence
- vesicoureteric reflux and hydronephrosis

Continued

- detrusor underactivity with inefficient voiding (low-pressure, low-flow voiding)
- raised postvoid residual
- compensatory abdominal straining during voiding
- small, 'spherical' bladder on screening.

Urodynamics following cystoplasty

Enterocystoplasty is a major operative treatment for bladder dysfunction such as intractable detrusor overactivity, painful bladder syndrome/interstitial cystitis, post-irradiation fibrosis, post–ketamine abuse bladder and tuberculosis. During this procedure the bladder is opened as in clam cystoplasty, and a small or large bowel segment is opened (detubularized) and patched onto the bladder. This serves to increase the bladder capacity.

All patients for whom such a procedure is planned should undergo careful urodynamic evaluation before the operation to establish a baseline for detrusor and bladder outlet function, to predict postprocedure complications and to exclude any other causes for the lower urinary tract symptoms.

Following cystoplasty, bowel peristalsis in the segment patched to the bladder frequently occurs and voiding is usually accomplished by abdominal straining, which is more efficient when coordinated with the peristaltic contractions. Unfortunately, some patients experience persistent or new symptoms such as urgency, daytime frequency, incontinence, voiding difficulty or recurrent urinary tract infections. Video urodynamics is important in the evaluation of post-cystoplasty problems, and attention should be paid to several important factors:

- Is the cystoplasty overactive?
- Is this overactivity associated with outflow obstruction?
- Is incontinence due to hyperactivity of the bowel segment or impaired outflow resistance?
- PVR should also be measured, usually by ultrasound bladder scanning.
- Are the continuing symptoms due to persistence of the underlying sensory bladder problem, where cystectomy and another form of cystoplasty or diversion may be appropriate?

Management

Overactive cystoplasties associated with outflow obstruction are best treated by first relieving the obstruction:

- in females, this usually means urethral dilatation
- in males, bladder neck incision or transurethral prostatectomy may be indicated.

Overactive cystoplasties without obstruction are best treated by pharmaco-therapy initially. Anticholinergic therapy is usually used, as are antispas-modic drugs such as mebeverine, although drug therapy may not be successful. If drug therapy fails, a further detubularization procedure to add a patch of small bowel to the side of the cystoplasty may be helpful; this reduces the activity of the cystoplasty and allows many patients, particularly females, to void to completion by abdominal straining and thereby minimise adverse symptoms. However, underactive cystoplasties can be associated with a large PVR, which in turn can lead to recurrent urinary tract infections. This problem is more likely to occur in males, in whom outflow resistance is higher and where abdominal straining is less efficient; in such cases, clean intermittent self-catheterization may be required.

CHAPTER 9

Neurogenic bladder disorders

INTRODUCTION

Neurogenic bladder dysfunction describes abnormal function of the bladder and urethra due to lesions affecting their innervation, either within the central nervous system or in the peripheral nerves of the lower urinary tract.

Neurological conditions can alter bladder and urethral function by altering:

- detrusor function
- striated muscle sphincter activity
- smooth muscle sphincter activity
- bladder and urethral sensation.

PATTERNS OF NEUROGENIC DYSFUNCTION

Although each individual patient will have a unique pattern of lower urinary tract dysfunction and require an individual management plan, the site of the lesion gives an indication of the likely pattern of the dysfunction.

Neurological lesions can be divided into four broad anatomical areas:

1. suprapontine
2. pontine (brainstem)
3. suprasacral spinal cord
4. sacral–subsacral (peripheral nerve and cauda equina).

Suprapontine

Causes – Suprapontine disorders typically are due to cerebrovascular accidents, brain tumours, head injury, dementia and cerebral palsy.

Pattern of dysfunction – Neurogenic detrusor overactivity (NDO) commonly occurs due to reduced cortical inhibitory control of the micturition

165

reflex. As the pontine coordination centres are unaffected by this lesion, detrusor and sphincter function coordination are preserved; for this reason, patients with suprapontine lesions usually do not develop high-pressure neurogenic bladders. However, many patients appropriately increase sphincter activity during detrusor overactivity to avoid urgency incontinence, and this increase in electromyography (EMG) activity has been termed *pseudodyssynergia*. In addition, some patients with cortical lesions lose the ability to voluntarily void, whilst others lose the sensation of bladder fullness and urgency.

Pontine

Causes – Pontine disorders typically are due to Parkinson's disease, multiple system atrophy and multiple sclerosis (MS).

Pattern of dysfunction – The brainstem contains both the pontine micturition centre and the pontine storage centre, and therefore a lesion in this area can cause of variety of storage and voiding dysfunctions to occur simultaneously. These include NDO, detrusor underactivity, detrusor sphincter dyssynergia (DSD) and external sphincter relaxation.

Suprasacral spinal cord

Causes – Suprasacral spinal cord disorders typically are due to spinal cord injury (SCI) and MS.

Pattern of dysfunction – Due to the loss of higher detrusor inhibition and coordination of voiding, these patients typically have detrusor overactivity associated with DSD. Bladder filling sensation will also be lost in a complete SCI. Spontaneous reflex voiding can occur; however, it is uncontrolled and associated with incontinence. DSD may lead to high voiding pressure and upper tract damage, and this is a particularly 'dangerous' pattern of urological dysfunction; it is typically seen in high-level (cervical cord) lesions.

Sacral and subsacral

Causes – These typically result from myelomeningocoele, spina bifida, MS and diabetes mellitus or are iatrogenic from surgical injury.

Pattern of dysfunction – A variety of patterns of dysfunction are seen depending on the level of the lesion and the extent of the denervation.

A complete sacral or subsacral lesion will lead to an acontractile detrusor, incompetent urethra and loss of bladder sensation. A complete lesion around the conus may demonstrate an acontractile detrusor with a normal or overactive urethra. A complete lumbosacral lesion may cause an overactive detrusor with an incompetent urethra. However, most lesions are incomplete and, depending on the pathways disrupted, can give a varying pattern of dysfunction. For example, injury to the pudendal nerves may lead to an incompetent urethra, whilst an injury to the pelvic nerves may lead to an underactive detrusor with impaired bladder sensation but with a normally functioning urethra. Injury to the afferent axons and pathways may lead to diminished bladder sensation. In addition, incomplete lesions can result in NDO and high-pressure neurogenic bladders.

URODYNAMICS FOR NEUROGENIC BLADDER DISORDERS

In the management of neurogenic lower urinary tract function, there are two goals.
- The primary aim is to protect the upper urinary tract:
  - ○ to maintain low intravesical pressures
  - ○ to maintain a low postvoid residual.
- The secondary aims are to improve the quality of life and/or achieve continence.

Urodynamic investigations can characterize the nature of the detrusor and sphincteric abnormality to:
- identify those patients who are at risk of upper tract damage
- formulate the best treatment strategies to achieve efficient bladder emptying and continence and reduce the incidence of urinary tract infections and autonomic dysreflexia.

Many patients with neurological disorders do not display symptoms or signs until significant damage has occurred to the upper tracts or to detrusor function. Urodynamic findings in this group of patients frequently do not correlate well with the neurological examination findings, and therefore the examination findings should not be used to plan the urological management. Instead, all patients with neurological dysfunction that affects or is likely to affect lower urinary tract function should receive a thorough urodynamic assessment at an early stage to fully characterize the function and to plan appropriate management; patients may require subsequent follow-up urodynamic investigations to determine the success of any intervention and the extent of any change in lower urinary tract function.

167

Assessment of lower urinary tract dysfunction is no different from that in neurologically normal patients, consisting of history, examination, voiding diaries, uroflowmetry and pressure/flow studies (± EMG). However, the interpretation is often more complex, and there are specific hazards such as autonomic dysreflexia; therefore the investigations are best performed in specialist centres using video urodynamics. It must be remembered that patients with neurogenic bladder dysfunction also suffer from the same lower urinary tract disorders as the rest of the population (e.g. bladder outflow obstruction related to the prostate), and these conditions may further complicate assessment and management. Management should be tailored for each patient depending on the pattern of dysfunction and a plan for follow-up, other relevant investigations (renal function, ultrasound) and repeat urodynamic assessments should be carried out.

NEUROGENIC DETRUSOR AND SPHINCTER OVERACTIVITY

The presence of both NDO and sphincter overactivity is a particularly dangerous urodynamic situation. As a rule of thumb, those patients with a competent bladder outflow and a pre-micturition pressure of 40 cm H_2O or higher are particularly at risk of developing upper urinary tract problems due to the high backpressure, although this is by no means an absolute value, and damage to the upper tracts can occur at lower pressures (Fig. 9.1).

Fig. 9.1 *Video urodynamic screening in a patient with spinal cord injury.*
Obstruction at the level of the sphincter (detrusor sphincter dyssynergia), right vesicoureteric reflux and hydronephrosis, as well as multiple bladder diverticulae, are seen.

If this pattern of dysfunction is present, then the preservation of renal function is of the utmost importance; this requires control of both NDO and sphincter overactivity.

Treatment strategies for NDO include:

- anticholinergics
- botulinum toxin therapy to the bladder
- neuromodulation
- bladder surgery (i.e. augmentation).

Treatment strategies for the overactive sphincter are to ensure adequate drainage; these include:

- clean intermittent self-catheterization
- botulinum toxin therapy to the sphincter
- neuromodulation
- sphincterotomy.

Incontinence that occurs as a result of a sphincterotomy can be controlled by implanting an artificial urinary sphincter.

The patient should at least have annual urodynamic assessments, postvoid residual and kidney function tests performed and should be followed up according to recognized guidelines, such as those produced by the International Consultation on Incontinence (ICI).

SPINAL SHOCK

Patients who have lesions above the sacral micturition centre initially go through a period of spinal shock in which there is loss of neurological (reflex) activity below the level of the injury. This usually results in complete urinary retention due to an acontractile detrusor and also to the maintenance of some residual sphincteric competence. Until there is recovery of some neurological activity, the patient will require either indwelling or intermittent catheterization.

URODYNAMICS IN PRACTICE: NEUROGENIC BLADDER DYSFUNCTION

- Initial urodynamic studies are most commonly performed after the spinal shock period is over (usually 3–4 months after spinal cord injury) when reflex activity is reestablished, along with a baseline renal ultrasound or intravenous urography.
- Routine urodynamics and renal radiography are usually performed annually or every alternate year depending on the nature of the vesicourethral dysfunction.

Continued

- Indications for nonroutine urodynamic investigation in patients with neurogenic disorders include symptomatic voiding dysfunction, urinary incontinence, renal deterioration (e.g. renal scarring, hydronephrosis, elevated serum creatinine level), recurrent urinary tract infections, a change in voiding pattern and the onset of autonomic dysreflexia.

Technique

- Many authorities recommend not emptying the bladder before commencing filling cystometry in patients who have NDO, because these patients usually have persistently high postvoid residuals and rapid bladder evacuation may alter the characteristics of the detrusor overactivity, resulting in an overdiagnosis of poor bladder compliance.
- Residual urine estimation by catheter or ultrasound should be carried out at another time, when emptying is more physiological.
- Some patients improve emptying during urodynamics by abdominal straining, suprapubic compression or triggering reflex detrusor contractions by perineal or abdominal tapping.
- The filling rate should be slow to not provoke premature detrusor overactivity, which may potentially mask information regarding sensations, cystometric capacity and compliance. Rapid filling may also trigger detrusor sphincter dyssynergia and overdiagnose poor bladder compliance. In addition, 30 seconds at the end of filling should be allowed for bladder accommodation before interpreting the pre-micturition pressure.
- Observation of several filling–voiding cycles is recommended to accurately define bladder and urethral abnormalities – the first voiding sequence may be altered by passing the catheter, which may precipitate or inhibit detrusor overactivity and be unrepresentative of the established pattern; suprapubic catheterization may eliminate this problem and is routinely used by some spinal injury centres.
- Symptomatic urinary tract infections alter urodynamic results and should be treated before urodynamic evaluation. Asymptomatic bacteriuria is common and predisposes patients to bacteraemia; it is recommended to use antibiotics 1 hour before the study if necessary.
- Video urodynamics provides the gold standard evaluation of patients who have neurogenic bladder dysfunction. It has the advantage of pressure/flow cystometry whilst allowing simultaneous anatomical visualization of the bladder and urethra, thus providing information about bladder size and shape, the presence of vesicoureteric reflux, the competency of the bladder neck and the site of bladder outflow obstruction. Video urodynamics reduces the importance of simultaneous electromyography for diagnosing detrusor sphincter dyssynergia.

PRACTICAL POINTS IN PERFORMING PRESSURE/FLOW CYSTOMETRY

Performing urodynamics in patients who have neurogenic bladder dysfunction can be challenging, and technical modifications may be necessary to obtain the maximum amount of information. Specific issues include:

- Paralysed patients are unable to stand and are best studied in the supine oblique position to obtain maximal visualization of the bladder neck and urethra.
- Voided urine can be transferred from the patient to the flowmeter using a length of guttering, which in male patients is fixed to the penis and thigh with tape.
- Sudden bursts of leg or abdominal spasms are not uncommon and may precede detrusor contractions or result in loss of the recording catheters.
- Rectal impaction can theoretically alter vesicoureteric function during urodynamic evaluation, and rectal evacuation before the study is therefore advised. If suppositories or rectal solutions are used, urodynamics should be delayed until there is a bowel action. Rectal catheterization commonly stimulates bowel evacuation in patients who have an SCI.
- Transurethral catheterization may be difficult in patients who have suprasacral cord lesions because of sphincter spasm.
- Autonomic dysreflexia is a specific risk in this population (see later discussion).

Detrusor leak point pressure

In neurogenic patients who have a high filling pressure, the upper tracts have an increased risk of being damaged if there is a subtracted detrusor pressure greater than 30–40 cm H_2O documented during filling cystometry. It is important to realize that neurogenic patients can have dangerously high detrusor leak point pressures, even though they have stress urinary incontinence and low abdominal leak point pressures secondary to intrinsic sphincter deficiency (see Chapter 4).

Autonomic dysreflexia

Autonomic dysreflexia is the exaggerated sympathetic output that occurs in response to a noxious autonomic stimulus below the level of injury in patients who have SCIs above T6. This manifests as hypertension associated with bradycardia, headache, profuse sweating and flushing above the level of the injury. Spontaneous bladder overdistension or high detrusor pressures may precipitate episodes of autonomic dysreflexia and may be due to a blocked catheter, inadequate drainage, bladder stones or urinary tract infection. Similarly, pressure/flow cystometry may also precipitate autonomic dysreflexia during filling or in relation to DSD and should be prevented by slow filling rates and the maintenance of low volumes and detrusor pressures. Autonomic dysreflexia is a life-threatening event and must be treated immediately. All units performing urodynamics on patients with SCIs should have a protocol in place for emergency treatment of the condition.

If autonomic dysreflexia occurs during pressure/flow urodynamics:

- Stop filling and empty the bladder as soon as possible with a large urethral catheter.
- Sit the patient up/raise the head.
- Loosen/remove any tight-fitting or constrictive clothing.
- Measure the blood pressure.
- Administer sublingual nifedipine 10 mg to lower the blood pressure rapidly if this remains greater than 150 mmHg despite the preceding steps.
- Continue treatment and regular blood pressure monitoring as per local guidelines.

ELECTROMYOGRAPHY

EMG (see Chapter 3) is the study of the bioelectric potentials generated by depolarization of skeletal muscle. The primary value of EMG is for identifying neuropathy. The functional unit in EMG is the motor unit, which is composed of:

- a varying number of muscle fibres supplied by the same motor neurone
- the axon of the motor neurone.

An excitatory impulse in the motor neurone causes each of its muscle fibres to contract; the sum of this activity is called the *motor unit action potential* (MUAP). The waveform of the MUAP is generally biphasic or triphasic and may be detected by electrodes and displayed on an oscilloscope screen or a strip chart, or on a urodynamic monitor if performed synchronously with pressure/flow cystometry.

Individually recorded on an oscilloscope, the MUAP has its own amplitude, duration and firing frequency. When a motor neurone is damaged, the muscle fibres that have lost their nerve supply become reinnervated by adjacent healthy nerve fibres, resulting in fewer but larger motor units. This results in MUAPs of larger amplitude and increased complexity (polyphasic) and duration. These changes in EMG may be used to infer the presence of neurological disease.

Types of electrode

Surface electrodes

Surface electrodes (skin, anal plug and catheter) record total electrical output from the muscles of the pelvic floor and are the standard electrodes used in clinical practice. They cannot record individual MUAPs, but they do allow assessment of overall muscle behaviour. Surface electrodes should be applied to an area as close to the muscle under investigation as possible. They can be difficult to secure and provide less reproducible results than needle electrodes.

Needle electrodes

Individual MUAPs may be detected by needle electrodes placed directly into or near the muscle to be studied. The needle most commonly is placed directly into the periurethral sphincter. A variety of different types of needle electrodes exist, including concentric, bipolar, monopolar and single fibre. They permit a more precise recording of EMG activity and analysis of individual MUAPs than surface electrodes. However, the technique is user dependent and requires considerable expertise; it is also uncomfortable for patients. Its use is therefore generally limited to research and highly specialized centres.

Recording site

EMGs are commonly recorded from three muscles:
1. the external anal sphincter
2. the levator ani
3. the striated urethral sphincter.

The easiest muscle to use is the external anal sphincter because placement is simple and dislodgement is less common. In most patients the EMG recorded from the three sites is similar, but in some neurological disorders, particularly demyelinating disease and partial cauda equina lesions, there may be significant differences between the recordings. It is therefore recommended by many to always record from the periurethral musculature.

Interpretation

Volitional control of the urinary sphincter is demonstrated by an increase and decrease in EMG activity associated with active contraction and relaxation of the pelvic floor musculature, respectively.

During filling, there is a normal progressive increase in EMG activity, which is referred to as recruitment. Just prior to voiding, the urethral musculature should relax and electrical silence during EMG monitoring is seen (Appendix 3, example trace 1). This relaxation should persist throughout the detrusor contraction.

Abnormal persistent EMG activity during voiding can be due to:
- the fact that complete electrical silence does not always occur
- straining artefact
- DSD
- pelvic floor dyssynergia (Appendix 3, example trace 5).

In contrast, pseudodyssynergia is the normal voluntary contraction of the external sphincter and pelvic floor muscles in response to an involuntary detrusor contraction (in the filling phase of the study) in an attempt to prevent urgency incontinence.

True DSD occurs only in patients who have neurological disorders. Several patterns of DSD have been described on EMG:
- a crescendo increase in EMG activity that reaches a peak at the peak of the detrusor contraction
- alternating contraction and relaxation (clonic EMG activity) of the sphincter musculature during the detrusor contraction (Appendix 3, example trace 4)
- sustained sphincter contraction throughout the period of the contraction (failure of relaxation).

OTHER SPECIALIZED NEUROPHYSIOLOGICAL STUDIES

Nerve conduction studies

These are performed by stimulating a peripheral nerve and monitoring the time for a response to occur in its innervated muscle. The time until the first measurable muscle response is termed *motor latency*. These studies test the integrity of nerve pathways, demonstrating prolonged latencies when there is injury to the nerve with associated demyelination.

The most commonly tested latency used to assess neuropathic bladder dysfunction is the bulbocavernosus reflex.

Nerve conduction studies have been found to be beneficial in diagnosing neurological disease but require elaborate instrumentation and expert interpretation.

Evoked responses

Evoked responses are potential changes in neural tissue resulting from distant stimulation, usually electrical. They are used to test the integrity of peripheral, spinal and central nervous pathways. As with nerve conduction studies, their use is confined to specialized neurophysiology centres.

Bethanechol supersensitivity test

When an organ is deprived of its nerve supply, it will develop hypersensitivity to its own neurotransmitter (Cannon's law of denervation). The bethanechol supersensitivity test is based on this theory; during the test, 2.5 mg of bethanechol chloride, an acetylcholine-like agent, is administered subcutaneously following an initial pressure/flow study. During a repeat pressure/flow study, a rise in detrusor pressure greater than 15 cm H_2O compared to the first study at 100-mL filling is a positive result and implies that the detrusor is denervated. A negative result suggests that the detrusor underactivity is due to a nonneurological cause.

False-negative and false-positive results are common, and bethanechol is contraindicated in patients who have cardiac disease, hypertension, asthma, peptic ulcer or bladder outflow obstruction. The use of this technique remains contentious.

Ice water test

Cold temperature provokes the bladder and increases detrusor activity. The ice water test is performed by instilling 90 mL of sterile ice-cold water (4°C) into an empty bladder through a 16-French catheter without filling the catheter balloon. The test is positive if the catheter is ejected together with a significant amount of water within 1 minute of installation (in the absence of straining). A positive result implies that the patient has NDO and may be of some use in diagnosing the cause of incontinence in patients with an SCI (Fig. 9.2).

175

Fig. 9.2 **Urodynamic trace.** *The trace shows neurogenic detrusor overactivity associated with an incompetent urethral mechanism. Note the relatively low voiding pressure and 'normal' flow rate.*

NEUROGENIC BLADDER DYSFUNCTION: PRACTICAL POINTS

- Detrusor sphincter dyssynergia is a pathognomonic feature of suprasacral spinal cord neurogenic bladder dysfunction.
- Several cystometric patterns are commonly seen in patients with neurogenic bladder:
  - ○ loss of bladder compliance
  - ○ high-pressure detrusor overactivity, often repetitive in a phasic 'systolic' pattern (Fig. 9.3a)
  - ○ detrusor overactivity in a 'stepping' pattern (consecutive detrusor contractions probably superimposed on loss of compliance) (Fig. 9.3b).
- Patients with neurogenic bladder may demonstrate a hyposensitive bladder or absent bladder sensation.
- Neurogenic patients may not be able to generate a voluntary detrusor contraction.
- Video urodynamics may demonstrate several abnormalities:
  - ○ bladder trabeculation and/or diverticula, or a 'Christmas tree'-shaped bladder
  - ○ vesicoureteral reflux
  - ○ decompensated bladder neck and/or prostatic urethra
  - ○ bladder neck and/or distal sphincter dyssynergia.

Fig. 9.3 *Patterns of detrusor overactivity frequently seen in neurogenic dysfunction.* (**a**) *Repetitive phasic detrusor contractions with a crescendo and stepping pattern as the bladder volume increases.* (**b**) *A stepping pattern with consecutive detrusor contractions. It is probable that there is also an underlying decrease in bladder compliance, with the detrusor contractions 'superimposed' on this.*

CHAPTER 10

Paediatric urodynamics

INTRODUCTION

Lower urinary tract dysfunction is common in children from both nonneurogenic and neurogenic causes. Most cases are well-recognized functional voiding disorders or have an underlying abnormality such as bladder outflow obstruction, and diagnosis does not depend on the use of urodynamics. As a general rule, urodynamics is not routinely required in the evaluation of nonneurogenic paediatric voiding dysfunction, as in most cases adequate diagnosis and treatment can be based on a thorough history and physical examination with appropriate use of endoscopy and radiography. However, urodynamic studies are important investigations in the evaluation and treatment of children with neurogenic bladder dysfunction, commonly due to spinal abnormalities.

Paediatric urodynamics is a highly specialized field and should only be performed in centres with the necessary equipment and expertise.

PAEDIATRIC LOWER URINARY TRACT DYSFUNCTION

As in adults, lower urinary tract dysfunction in children can be categorized as either storage or voiding. These include:

- storage:
  - incontinence:
    - urgency incontinence (most frequent)
    - overflow incontinence
    - other causes of incontinence
  - nocturnal enuresis (NE)
- voiding:
  - functional obstruction
  - mechanical obstruction.

Nocturnal enuresis is defined as the involuntary leakage of urine that occurs during sleep and in children is considered abnormal after the age of 5 years, with no other urinary tract dysfunction. NE can be mono-symptomatic or nonmonosymptomatic, where the condition is associated with other storage-type lower urinary tract symptoms. Urodynamic studies are generally not required in the assessment of NE, and most children with monosymptomatic NE become dry by age 10, whilst behavioural treatments including alarm systems can be useful in this group of patients. Nonmonosymptomatic NE can be associated with detrusor over-activity (DO), and therefore pharmacotherapies directed at the treatment of overactivity can result in symptomatic relief for both the daytime and nighttime component.

Incontinence may be due to several causes, and a urodynamic study may be helpful in determining the cause and planning the management. Mechanical obstruction in boys may be due to urethral valves, phimosis or meatal stenosis, and in girls it may be due to urethral stenosis. Functional obstruction is due to detrusor sphincter dyssynergia (DSD) secondary to a neurological abnormality or secondary to poor relaxation of the pelvic floor and urethral sphincter mechanism.

HISTORY AND EXAMINATION

Urodynamics is not required in most nonneurogenic childhood urinary tract dysfunction, and therefore a detailed history and physical examination is required to:
- characterize the bladder dysfunction
- identify underlying organic disease
- identify common functional voiding syndromes.

A detailed voiding history is essential and should include:
- age and results of toilet training
- occurrence of primary or secondary enuresis
- the specific pattern of wetting, such as stress incontinence, continual dripping or urge incontinence
- manoeuvres used to prevent wetting, such as squatting, leg crossing, dancing or 'Vincent's curtsy' (see later discussion)
- frequency of daytime and nighttime micturition.

Physical examination should include:
- inspection of the genitalia
- palpation of the lumbosacral spine to detect vertebral defects or sacral agenesis

- examination of the skin overlying the spine for hairy patches, dimples or bumps that might indicate occult spinal abnormalities
- inspection of the lower extremities for subtle neuropathy-related bony abnormalities
- a careful neurological examination.

Investigations should include:
- urinalysis
- postvoid residual estimation.

Functional disorders

Functional disorders often resolve spontaneously, and usually urodynamic studies add little to the diagnosis and treatment of these children and should be reserved for select cases. A common pattern is seen in 4- to 7-year-olds; symptoms commonly include frequency and urgency incontinence, yet bladder signals appear to be ignored during play activities. Girls may display the Vincent's curtsy sign, where the heel is pressed into the perineum to prevent incontinence secondary to detrusor contractions. Most cases resolve spontaneously, but some may require a period of anticholinergic medication to alleviate symptoms.

INDICATIONS FOR URODYNAMICS

Indications for urodynamic investigations in children include:
- suspected neurogenic dysfunction such as DSD
- voiding dysfunction associated with significant bladder hypertrophy, vesicoureteric reflux or upper urinary tract damage
- daytime incontinence that is troublesome for the child, refractory to conservative therapy and not typical of common functional voiding disorders
- symptomatic patients suspected of having occult neuropathy
- persistent NE and recurrent urinary tract infections in some children (rare).

URODYNAMIC INVESTIGATIONS

All urodynamic investigations in children require time, patience and, above all, experienced interpretation.

Uroflowmetry

In general the usefulness of uroflowmetry in the evaluation of paediatric voiding dysfunction is limited because flow rates vary with age, sex and volume voided, preventing the establishment of standard values. The child must be old enough to follow instructions and void in his or her usual fashion; often a normal pattern associated with efficient bladder emptying may be sufficient, making further urodynamic testing unnecessary. Measurement of the postvoid residual urine volume with a bladder scanner remains an important part of the clinical evaluation.

Electromyography

Electromyography (EMG) of the striated muscles of the pelvic floor is necessary to assess the synergy between the bladder and urethral sphincter mechanisms during voiding. Uroflowmetry with simultaneous EMG is frequently performed in children and may help differentiate DSD from abdominal straining during voiding. The EMG electrodes can be placed on the pelvic floor or on the abdominal muscles. Increased EMG activity secondary to straining is common in children and must be differentiated from true DSD, which is diagnostic of neurogenic bladder dysfunction.

EMG is also usually performed concurrently with cystometry (see the next section). Surface patch electrodes are used in most cases, but fine needle electrodes placed directly into the periurethral striated sphincter are recommended to diagnose neuropathy; however, this is not normally feasible in children.

Cystometry

Filling using 5 to 8 French urethral catheters or feeding tubes is recommended. Filling can be performed transurethrally or in select cases using lines that have been suprapubically inserted under anaesthesia. The suprapubic line should have been in at least 6 hours, although a much longer period prior to performing the study is preferable.

The rectal catheter and EMG surface electrodes can be placed immediately before starting the investigation. If the rectal catheter is not well tolerated, abdominal wall EMG may be used to detect abdominal wall muscle activity, giving an indirect measure of abdominal pressure.

Infusion rates depend on the cystometric capacity, which is dependent on age. Adults are filled at a rate of approximately 10% of the bladder capacity (i.e. 50 mL/min for a 500-mL capacity bladder). Children should be filled at the same rate (10–25 mL/min); however, in neurogenic dysfunction the rate should be lowered even further. Bladder capacity in children can be calculated from the following formula:

$$\text{Age (years)} \times 30 + 30 = \text{bladder capacity (mL)}$$

The child can be filled while in a supine or sitting position and should be encouraged to void in a position and fashion that is as normal as possible. Children ideally should be fully awake during cystometry, but in some cases mild sedation is required to obtain useful information.

Video urodynamics

Video urodynamics provides a more comprehensive evaluation, especially in patients who have neurogenic bladder dysfunction, bladder outflow obstruction and incontinence.

DSD can be diagnosed during fluoroscopy without direct measurement of EMG activity, eliminating the need for potentially bothersome electrodes.

URODYNAMICS IN PRACTICE: PAEDIATRIC PATIENTS

- A urodynamic investigation is only useful if it can be performed without undue anxiety; patient cooperation allowing reproduction of the normal voiding pattern is of utmost importance to obtain useful clinical information.
- A pleasant, cheerful testing environment and staff and the presence of a family member will help reduce fear and anxiety.
- Common helpful distracters include movies, television, games, toys and favourite treats.

INTERPRETATION

Because of the great variability in the development of urinary control in young children, extreme caution is needed in interpreting their urodynamics and in diagnosing disorders of lower urinary tract function. Urodynamics must therefore not be undertaken lightly in this group and must be interpreted with care.

It is likely that all children transiently display abnormalities in bladder and sphincter function when making the transition from infantile to adult patterns of urinary control. Provided that these are not sustained, they do not appear to be pathological or to carry any long-term consequences.

As with adult pressure/flow studies, cystometry provides useful information about bladder capacity, sensation, compliance and detrusor/urethral function. The maximum cystometric capacity is often lower than the calculated anatomical capacity and depends on the child's ability to suppress voiding.

An estimation of bladder sensitivity (hypersensitive, hyposensitive or normal) can be made during filling. Filling is usually limited by:

- a sensation of bladder fullness or even pain
- urinary incontinence secondary to DO or poor detrusor compliance
- uncontrollable spontaneous voiding.

Detrusor overactivity – DO may or may not represent a clinically significant abnormality, depending on the child's age and voluntary response to the overactivity. Overactive contractions are considered to be normal in young immature bladders until central inhibitory pathways develop fully, even in the face of a strong desire to void. This maturation usually occurs by 4 years of age and often much earlier. Prior to maturation, voiding is involuntary and usually to completion, as a result of a well-sustained detrusor contraction accompanied by synergic relaxation of the urethral sphincter mechanism.

Dysfunctional voiding – Voluntary contraction of the external sphincter in an attempt to prevent incontinence is common in the early development of normal urinary control. This results in an obstruction to flow with high intravesical pressure. In some children, this 'voluntary dyssynergia' can remain, resulting in long-term voiding dysfunction. Renal damage can result in the most severe of cases. This pattern of dysfunctional voiding is known as Hinman's syndrome and was previously termed *nonneuropathic neuropathic bladder*.

Detrusor sphincter dyssynergia – Voluntary contraction of the external sphincter to prevent leakage during involuntary detrusor contractions is commonly misinterpreted as DSD in patients who do not have neuropathy. This is an appropriate patient response in an attempt to maintain continence and can be referred to as pseudodyssynergia. To make the important distinction between DSD and pseudodyssynergia, the patient should be asked to void voluntarily. During DSD, continued EMG activity in the external sphincter will occur, whilst in pseudodyssynergia the EMG activity should become silent.

Compliance – Reduced bladder compliance is commonly found in children who have neurogenic bladder dysfunction. The pre-micturition pressure is normally less than 10 cm H_2O. Children who have myelomeningocoele and reduced bladder compliance with a detrusor leak point pressure greater than 40 cm H_2O are at risk of renal damage as a result of the high detrusor pressure.

Scheme for performing a pressure/flow study

In this appendix a scheme for performing a pressure/flow study is summarized. It is good practice to perform urodynamics in a standard routine to ensure that all possible data are obtained. However, each individual study should be modified to ensure that the urodynamic question and other relevant data are fully obtained without undue effort being spent obtaining clinically irrelevant data. In addition, the scheme should be modified depending on local facilities.

PRIOR TO THE TEST: PATIENT FACTORS

- Reassess clinical history and the 'urodynamic question'.
- Perform physical examination if necessary.
- Obtain consent for procedure.
- Assess voiding diary to determine bladder capacity at which to stop filling (if not previously done).
- Identify whether medications which could influence the study findings have been discontinued.
- Perform initial free uroflowmetry for comparison and quality control (if not previously done).
- Exclude urinary tract infection (urinalysis).
- Consider if prophylactic antibiotics are necessary.

PRIOR TO THE TEST: EQUIPMENT FACTORS AND SETUP

- Ensure that equipment is calibrated, set up correctly and functioning.
- Insert intravesical measuring and filling lines with the patient in the supine position using an aseptic technique (and lidocaine gel in men).
- Insert an intraabdominal measuring line with the patient in the left lateral position; ensure that a slit is cut in the rectal balloon.

- Drain the bladder to assess the initial residual urine or fill on top of the initial residual and calculate the initial residual later.
- Connect catheters to the transducers/recording equipment and the filling pump.
- Flush fluid lines, and ensure that all air bubbles from both the tubing and transducer chambers have been excluded.
- Zero to atmospheric pressure (perform this prior to catheter insertion if using microtip catheters).
- Set the reference height to the level of the pubic symphysis.
- Ensure that resting values are within the expected range.
- Ensure that no dampening is present.

STARTING THE TEST

- Begin recording.
- Perform a quality control cough and repeat every 1 minute (and before and after any events).
- Start filling at the desired rate.
- Adjust patient position; standing is preferable (many urodynamicists stand the patient when the first sensation of filling occurs).
- Adjust the reference height with each change of patient position.
- Maintain constant interaction with the patient.
- Monitor the intraabdominal, intravesical and subtracted detrusor traces throughout the study.

STORAGE PHASE

- Ensure that the patient is trying to suppress voiding/leakage during the storage phase.
- Record the volume of the first sensation of filling, first desire to void and strong desire to void.
- Record any episodes of urgency and/or leakage.
- Assess for stress incontinence with intermittent coughs/Valsalva manoeuvre (in the oblique position if using video screening or with the patient lying flat with legs abducted or standing with legs slightly apart if screening is not available).
- Perform leak point pressure measurements if desired.
- Determine bladder compliance.
- Record episodes of detrusor overactivity, including the volume at which they occur, maximum rise in pressure and any associated urgency/leakage.
- Record the maximum cystometric capacity.

186

- Perform provocation tests at maximum cystometric capacity if detrusor overactivity was not detected previously.
- Use screening (if performing video urodynamics) to assess the bladder outline, volume, vesicoureteric reflux, diverticula, trabeculations, opening of the bladder neck, bladder neck descent, bladder neck hyper-mobility and leakage.
- Characterize the bladder and urethral function during the storage phase.

VOIDING PHASE

- Ensure that the patient coughs prior to voiding.
- Record the pre-micturition pressure.
- Allow the patient to void.
- Use screening to outline the urethra and determine the site of any obstruction, completeness of emptying and presence of any vesicoureteric reflux.
- Perform the stop test if desired.
- On completion of voiding, ensure that the patient coughs again.
- Adjust the flow trace for flow rate delay.
- Record voiding parameters, including maximum detrusor pressure, maximum flow rate, detrusor pressure at maximum flow rate and volume voided.
- Assess residual urine (and calculate the initial residual if necessary).
- Assess for bladder outflow obstruction ($P_{det}@Q_{max} - 2Q_{max}$) and the bladder outflow obstruction index ($P_{det}@Q_{max} + 5Q_{max}$).
- Characterize the bladder and urethral function during the voiding phase.
- Consider urethral pressure profilometry if thought to be appropriate.

AT THE END OF THE STUDY

- Determine whether the study needs to be repeated.
- Complete the study pro forma if used.
- Discuss findings with the patient.
- Write a study report and plan for further investigation/management.
- Ensure that the data is printed and suitably archived electronically.

Normal urodynamic values

Some pertinent normal urodynamic values are listed in this appendix. These serve only as a guide; all urodynamic findings should be interpreted with knowledge of the history, physical examination and investigation results, as well as findings from other urodynamic investigations. No urodynamic findings should be considered in isolation, as this will invariably lead to an incorrect interpretation of the results.

PAD TESTING

With the 1-hour International Continence Society pad test, the upper limit (99% confidence limit) has been found to be 1.4 g/hour. (However, it may be as high as 2.1 g/hour in women who consider themselves continent.)

UROFLOWMETRY

Men younger than 40 years : Q_{max} >25 mL/s
Men older than 60 years   : Q_{max} >15 mL/s
Females   : Q_{max} >30–35 mL/s

PRESSURE/FLOW STUDIES

Storage

Maximum cystometric capacity (MCC) : 350–600 mL
Volume at first sensation   : approximately 50% of the MCC
Volume at normal desire   : approximately 75% of the MCC
Volume at strong desire   : approximately 90% of the MCC
Normal compliance   : >30 mL/cm H_2O

Voiding

Maximum detrusor pressure	: 25–60 cm H_2O
$P_{det}@Q_{max}$ in men	: 40–60 cm H_2O
$P_{det}@Q_{max}$ in females	: 20–40 cm H_2O
Postvoid residual	: <25 mL
Bladder outflow obstruction index (BOOI)	: >20 obstructed
BOOI	: 20–40 equivocal
BOOI	: <20 unobstructed
Bladder contractility index (BCI)	: >150 strong contractility
BCI	: 100–150 normal contractility
BCI	: <100 weak contractility

Leak point pressures and urethral pressure profilometry

(These values are not universally accepted and remain an area of dispute.)

- Abdominal leak point pressure (ALPP) >100 cm H_2O: suggests urethral hypermobility.
- ALPP <60 cm H_2O: suggests intrinsic sphincter deficiency (ISD).
- Detrusor leak point pressure (DLPP) >40 cm H_2O: suggests upper tract deterioration likely.
- Maximum urethral closure pressure <20 cm H_2O: suggests ISD.

Example traces

	Storage phase	Voiding phase
Detrusor function	Normal, although rectal contractions give the misleading appearance of phasic detrusor overactivity	Overactive (high pressure)
Urethral/bladder outlet function	Normal; increased EMG activity due to rectal contractions and recruitment (see Chapter 9)	Prolonged, low flow (obstructive): appropriate decrease in EMG activity with voiding
Quality	Dampening of intravesical line, rectal contractions throughout, artefactual movements to flowmeter during storage phase	
Diagnosis	Bladder outflow obstruction	

Table A3.1   **EMG, Electromyography.**

	Storage phase	Voiding phase
Detrusor function	Detrusor overactivity following coughing	Not shown
Urethral/bladder outlet function	Urinary incontinence due to detrusor overactivity	Not shown
Quality	Acceptable	
Diagnosis	Cough-induced detrusor overactivity with incontinence	

Table A3.2

	Storage phase	Voiding phase
Detrusor function	Normal	High pressure (overactive)
Urethra/bladder outlet function	Normal	Low flow rate (<9 mL/s)
Quality	Subtraction appears acceptable, although no quality control coughs	
Diagnosis	Bladder outflow obstruction and superimposed screening image show a urethral stricture	

Table A3.3

	Storage phase	Voiding phase
Detrusor function	Overactive; recurrent contractions with 'stepping' pattern	High-pressure involuntary void (overactive)
Urethral/bladder outlet function	Competent	Intermittent flow with corresponding rises in detrusor pressure; electromyography shows intermittent sphincter activity
Quality	No quality control coughs, but subtraction appears acceptable	
Diagnosis	Neurogenic detrusor overactivity and detrusor sphincter dyssynergia	

Table A3.4

194

First sensation	925 mL infused volume
MCC	1182 mL infused volume
Q_{max}	29 mL/s
$P_{det}@Q_{max}$	24 cm H_2O
Voided volume	585 mL

195

	Storage phase	Voiding phase
Detrusor function	Hyposensitive with late first sensation at 925-mL filling and large cystometric capacity of 1182 mL	Low pressure ($P_{det}@Q_{max} = 24$ cm H_2O)
Urethra/bladder outlet function	Competent	Normal peak flow (29 mL/s), incomplete emptying (voided only 585 mL); increased EMG activity during voiding
Quality	Acceptable	
Diagnosis	Hyposensitive, large-capacity bladder. Possibly low detrusor pressure secondary to overdistension or developing poor detrusor contractility (detrusor underactivity). Increased EMG activity is compatible with detrusor sphincter dyssynergia or pelvic floor dyssynergia.	

Table A3.5 **EMG, *Electromyography.***

	Storage phase	Voiding phase
Detrusor function	Normal	Low-pressure void associated with abdominal straining
Urethral/bladder outlet function	Competent	Low flow rate with incomplete emptying; increased electromyography activity compatible with abdominal straining
Quality	Acceptable	
Diagnosis	Poor detrusor contractility (detrusor underactivity)	

Table A3.6

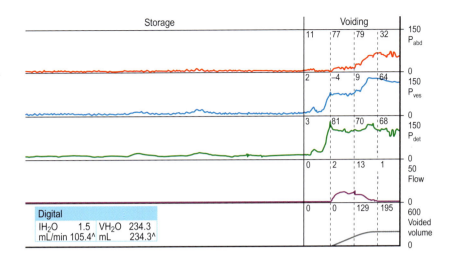

	Storage phase	Voiding phase
Detrusor function	Overactive	High pressure, although the subtraction does not appear to be accurate
Urethral/bladder outlet function	Competent	Low flow rate with additional abdominal straining
Quality	Quality control coughs not present, poor subtraction during voiding phase	
Diagnosis	Bladder outflow obstruction and detrusor overactivity	

Table A3.7

	Storage phase	Voiding phase
Detrusor function	Phasic detrusor overactivity	High pressure
Urethral/bladder outlet function	Leakage associated with detrusor overactivity	Low flow rate
Quality	Few quality control coughs, intraabdominal line dampening	
Diagnosis	Gross detrusor overactivity with incontinence, unable to interpret the voiding phase since void is initiated during a terminal contraction; the appearance of obstruction in this case may be due to the abnormally high pressures present at the start of voiding. The patient should have the voiding phase repeated to accurately define the voiding function.	

Table A3.8

	Storage phase	Voiding phase
Detrusor function	Overactive	High pressure
Urethral/bladder outlet function	Competent	Intermittent low flow rate with incomplete emptying and prostatic obstruction visible on screening image
Quality	Dampening in abdominal line; no coughs	
Diagnosis	Detrusor overactivity and bladder outflow obstruction secondary to prostatic obstruction	

Table A3.9

	Storage phase	Voiding phase
Detrusor function	Overactive and oversensitive with first sensation at 61-mL filling and MCC at 116-mL filling. Possible overactivity, but poor subtraction makes identification difficult.	Uninterpretable due to loss of urethral catheter
Urethral/ bladder outlet function	Competent	Poor flow with some abdominal straining
Quality	Dampening in abdominal line throughout study. Intravesical catheter voided out at the beginning of the voiding phase.	
Diagnosis	Oversensitivity and possible detrusor overactivity. Study needs to be repeated to determine detrusor function during voiding and storage phases with better quality control.	

Table A3.10

	Storage phase	Voiding phase
Detrusor function	Overactive	Normal pressure (P_{det} falsely elevated at end of filling due to drop in rectal pressure; voiding pressure appears normal based on P_{ves})
Urethral/bladder outlet function	Competent	Normal flow pattern, slightly low Q_{max}; need to perform free uroflowmetry to determine Q_{max} without an in situ catheter
Quality	High P_{abd} at baseline causing a negative detrusor pressure. Dampening of intraabdominal line throughout study. Immediately prior to voiding the patient changed position to sitting with no alteration in reference height. Poor-quality assessment.	
Diagnosis	Detrusor overactivity	

Table A3.11

	Storage phase	Voiding phase
Detrusor function	Normal	Uninterpretable due to loss of intraabdominal line, although possibly poor detrusor contractility
Urethral/bladder outlet function	Competent	Poor flow
Quality	Intraabdominal catheter passed out at beginning of voiding	
Diagnosis	Study needs to be repeated to determine subtracted detrusor function during voiding once intraabdominal line is replaced.	

Table A3.12

	Storage phase	Voiding phase
Detrusor function	Rectal contractions only	Overactive (high pressure)
Urethral/bladder outlet function	Competent (flow readings are artefacts)	Negligible flow despite additional abdominal straining
Quality	Impaired subtraction throughout study noticeable on quality control coughs	
Diagnosis	High-pressure bladder outflow obstruction	

Table A3.13

	Storage phase	Voiding phase
Detrusor function	Early bladder sensations suggesting some oversensitivity	Severely hypocontractile, with a prolonged time before commencing any voiding; intermittent voiding with a negligible amount passed
Urethra/bladder outlet function	Competent	Low-pressure, low-flow voiding despite abdominal straining
Quality	Slight dampening in abdominal line throughout study. Intraabdominal pressure is artefactually negative during parts of the study, leading to artefactual rise in detrusor pressure.	
Diagnosis	Detrusor underactivity, possibly some oversensitivity (detrusor hypersensitivity impaired contractility)	

Table A3.14

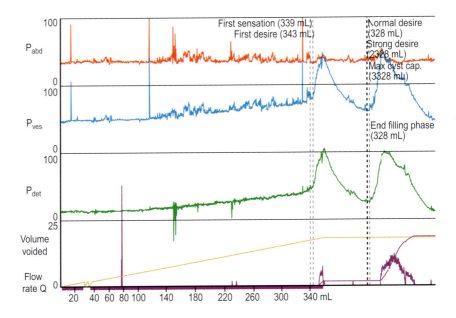

	Storage phase	Voiding phase
Detrusor function	Poor detrusor compliance; overactive with associated incontinence	No voluntary void; voided off an overactive contraction
Urethral/bladder outlet function	Leakage associated with detrusor overactivity	No voluntary void
Quality	Occasional dampening in intraabdominal line	
Diagnosis	Detrusor overactivity and poor bladder compliance	

Table A3.15

	Storage phase	Voiding phase
Detrusor function	Overactive, with several small involuntary contractions followed by a large terminal contraction; early sensations suggesting some oversensitivity	Voided during a terminal contraction
Urethral/bladder outlet function	Incompetent on coughing	Normal flow pattern
Quality	Dampening in abdominal line throughout study	
Diagnosis	Mixed incontinence, with some degree of oversensitivity; cannot interpret voiding phase, as voided off an overactive contraction	

Table A3.16

Bibliography

FURTHER READING

It is clear that urodynamic evaluation is essential to the accurate investigation of patients with lower urinary tract symptoms. As only a summary of this subject can be provided here, comprehensive reviews should be consulted for more detailed information:

Abrams P. *Urodynamics*. 3rd ed. London: Springer; 2006.

Abrams P, Cardozo L, Khoury S, Wein A. *Incontinence*. 5th ed. Paris: Health Publications; 2013.

The following are reports from the 5th International Consultation on Incontinence (also available online at http://www.icud.info/incontinence.html):

Mundy AR, Stephenson TP, Wein AJ. *Urodynamics: Principles, Practice and Application*. 2nd ed. Edinburgh: Churchill Livingstone; 1994.

Patel U. *Imaging and Urodynamics of the Lower Urinary Tract*. 2nd ed. London: Springer; 2010.

Wein AJ, Kavoussi LR, Partin AW, Peters CA. *Campbell-Walsh Urology*. 11th ed. Philadelphia: Elsevier; 2015.

INTERNATIONAL CONTINENCE SOCIETY DOCUMENTS AND REPORTS

The International Continence Society (ICS) has produced several standardization reports and documents regarding lower urinary tract dysfunction and investigation. These have been published widely and are also available on the ICS website (http://www.ics.org). Recent reports include:

Abrams P, Cardozo L, Fall M, et al. The standardisation of terminology in lower urinary tract function: report from the Standardisation Sub-Committee of the International Continence Society. *Urology*. 2003;61(1):37–49.

Austin PF, Bauer SB, Bower W, et al. The standardization of terminology of lower urinary tract function in children and adolescents: update report from the Standardization Committee of the International Children's Continence Society. *Neurourology and Urodynamics*. 2016;35(4):471–481.

Doggweiler R, Whitmore KE, Meijlink JM, et al. A standard for terminology in chronic pelvic pain syndromes: a report from the Chronic Pelvic Pain Working Group of the International Continence Society. *Neurourology and Urodynamics*. 2017;36(4):984–1008.

Griffiths D, Hofner K, van Mastrigt R, et al. Standardization of terminology of lower urinary tract function: pressure–flow studies of voiding, urethral resistance, and urethral obstruction. International Continence Society Subcommittee on Standardization of Terminology of Pressure–Flow Studies. *Neurourology and Urodynamics*. 1997;16(1):1–18.

Lose G, Griffiths D, Hosker G, et al. Standardisation of urethral pressure measurement: report from the Standardisation Sub-Committee of the International Continence Society. *Neurourology and Urodynamics*. 2002;21(3):258–260.

Messelink B, Benson T, Berghmans B, et al. Standardization of terminology of pelvic floor muscle function and dysfunction: report from the Pelvic Floor Clinical Assessment Group of the International Continence Society. *Neurourology and Urodynamics*. 2005;24(4):374–380.

Rosier PF, Schaefer W, Lose G, et al. International Continence Society Good Urodynamic Practices and Terms 2016: Urodynamics, uroflowmetry, cystometry, and pressure-flow study. *Neurourology and Urodynamics*. 2017;36(5):1243–1260.

Schafer W, Abrams P, Liao L, et al. Good urodynamic practices: uroflowmetry, filling cystometry, and pressure–flow studies. *Neurourology and Urodynamics*. 2002;21(3):261–274.

Stohrer M, Goepel M, Kondo A, et al. The standardization of terminology in neurogenic lower urinary tract dysfunction: with suggestions for diagnostic procedures. International Continence Society Standardization Committee. *Neurourology and Urodynamics*. 1999;18(2):139–158.

van Kerrebroeck P, Abrams P, Chaikin D, et al. The standardisation of terminology in nocturia: report from the Standardisation Sub-Committee of the International Continence Society. *Neurourology and Urodynamics*. 2002;21(2):179–183.

van Mastrigt R, Griffiths DJ. ICS standard for digital exchange of urodynamic study data. *Neurourology and Urodynamics*. 2004;23(3): 280–281.

van Waalwijk van Doorn E, Anders K, et al. Standardisation of ambulatory urodynamic monitoring: report of the Standardisation Sub-Committee of the International Continence Society for Ambulatory Urodynamic Studies. *Neurourology and Urodynamics*. 2000;19(2):113–125.

CLINICAL GUIDELINES

Clinical guidelines for the assessment and management of lower urinary tract disorders have been produced by several organizations, including:

- **American Urological Association (AUA):** http://www.auanet.org
- **European Association of Urology (EAU):** http://www.uroweb.org
- **International Consultation on Incontinence (ICI):** reports available at http://www.icud.info
- **International Consultation on Urological Diseases (ICUD),** such as the proceedings of the International Consultation on Benign Prostatic Hyperplasia
- **United Kingdom National Institute for Health and Clinical Excellence (NICE):** https://www.nice.org.uk

Up-to-date guidelines from these and other national and regional bodies should be consulted when assessing and managing patients with lower urinary tract dysfunction.

Index

Note: Page numbers followed by *f* indicate figures, *t* indicate tables, and *b* indicate boxes.

N

O

P